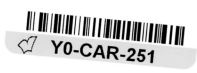

Retention and Stability in Orthodontics

Retention and Stability in Orthodontics

Ravindra Nanda, B.D.S., M.D.S., Ph.D.
Professor and Head
Division of Orthodontics
University of Connecticut
School of Dental Medicine
Farmington, Connecticut

Charles J. Burstone, D.D.S., M.S.
Professor
Division of Orthodontics
University of Connecticut
School of Dental Medicine
Farmington, Connecticut

W. B. SAUNDERS COMPANY
A Division of Harcourt, Brace & Company

Philadelphia / London / Toronto / Montreal / Sydney / Tokyo

W. B. SAUNDERS COMPANY

A Division of Harcourt, Brace & Company

The Curtis Center
Independence Square West
Philadelphia, PA 19106

Library of Congress Cataloging-in-Publication Data

Retention and stability in orthodontics / [edited by] Ravindra Nanda,
    Charles J. Burstone.
       p.   cm.
    ISBN 0–7216–4342–6
    1. Orthodontics—Complications.   2. Malocclusion—Relapse—Prevention.
  3. Teeth—Movements.   I. Nanda, Ravindra.   II. Burstone, Charles J.
    [DNLM: 1. Orthodontics, Corrective—methods.   2. Denture Retention.
  WU 400 R437 1993]
  RK527.4.R48   1993
  617.6'43—dc20
  DNLM/DLC

                                               93–10448

RETENTION AND STABILITY IN ORTHODONTICS   ISBN 0-7216-4342-6

Printed in the United States of America

Last digit is the print number: 9   8   7   6   5   4   3   2   1

To my wife,
Patti,
for her support and encouragement over the years.

and

To our *students,*
whose inquisitiveness has been
a continuing inspiration

CONTRIBUTORS

Richard G. Alexander, D.D.S., M.S.D.
Clinical Professor of Orthodontics, Baylor College of Dentistry, Waco, Texas
Treatment and Retention for Long-Term Stability

Charles J. Burstone, D.D.S., M.S.
Professor, Division of Orthodontics, School of Dental Medicine, University of Connecticut, Farmington, Connecticut
Perspectives in Orthodontic Stability

Jeffrey Burzin, D.D.S.
Private Practice, 674 Cove Road, Stamford, Connecticut, 06902
The Stability of Deep Overbite Correction

John C. Gorman, D.M.D., M.S.
Associate Professor, School of Dentistry, Indiana University, Bloomington, Indiana; Dental Staff, Marion General Hospital, Marion, Indiana
The Effects of Premolar Extractions on the Long-Term Stability of the Mandibular Incisors

Dietmar Kubein-Meesenburg, D.D.S.
Head, Department of Orthodontics, Universitat Göttingen, Göttingen, Germany
Biomechanical Aspects of Stability of Occlusion

Robert M. Little, D.D.S., M.S.D., Ph.D.
Professor and Graduate Program Director, Department of Orthodontics, School of Dentistry, University of Washington, Seattle, Washington
Stability and Relapse of Dental Arch Alignment

Hans Nägerl, Dr. med. habil.
Director, Physics Laboratory for Medical Students, Universitat Göttingen, Göttingen, Germany
Biomechanical Aspects of Stability of Occlusion

Ram S. Nanda, B.D.S., D.D.S., M.S., Ph.D.
Professor and Chairman, Department of Orthodontics; Chairman, Division of Developmental Dentistry, College of Dentistry; Adjunct Professor, Department of Anatomical Sciences, College of Medicine, University of Oklahoma, Oklahoma City, Oklahoma
Considerations of Dentofacial Growth in Long-Term Retention and Stability

Ravindra Nanda, B.D.S., M.D.S., Ph.D.
Professor and Head, Division of Orthodontics, School of Dental Medicine,
University of Connecticut, Farmington, Connecticut
Retention and Stability—An Overview
The Stability of Deep Overbite Correction

Surender K. Nanda, B.D.S., D.D.S., M.S.
Professor, Department of Orthodontics and Pediatric Dentistry, School of
Dentistry, University of Michigan, Ann Arbor, Michigan
Considerations of Dentofacial Growth in Long-Term Retention and Stability

Ib Leth Nielsen, D.D.S.
Clinical Professor, Department of Growth and Development, University of
California, San Francisco, California; Adjunct Professor, University of the
Pacific, School of Dentistry, San Francisco
Growth Considerations in Stability of Orthodontic Treatment

Cyril Sadowsky, D.D.S.
Professor of Orthodontics, College of Dentistry, University of Illinois at
Chicago, Chicago, Illinois
Long-Term Stability Following Orthodontic Therapy

Peter M. Sinclair, D.D.S., M.S.D.
Associate Professor, Head, Department of Orthodontics, University of
Southern California, Los Angeles, California
The Long-Term Stability of Orthognathic Surgery

Arthur T. Storey, D.D.S., M.S., Ph.D.
Professor and Chairman, Department of Orthodontics, Health Science
Center at San Antonio, University of Texas, San Antonio, Texas
*Functional Stability of Orthodontic Treatment—Occlusion as a Cause of
Temporomandibular Disorders*

Bjorn U. Zachrisson, D.D.S., M.S.D., Ph.D.
Professor II of Orthodontics, Dental Faculty, University of Oslo, Oslo,
Norway
Finishing and Retention Procedures for Improved Esthetics and Stability

Joseph Zernik, D.D.S., Ph.D.
Associate Professor, Department of Orthodontics, School of Dentistry,
University of Southern California, Los Angeles, California
Retention and Stability—An Overview

PREFACE

Long-term stability of achieved results is one of the major goals of orthodontic treatment. Some factors responsible for retention and stability, however, have not received as much attention as other areas, for example, diagnosis, treatment planning, and mechanics.

Over the years, numerous excellent books have been published in the field of orthodontics dealing with various phases of the specialty. This is the first book that brings together current and relevant knowledge to aid the clinician in achieving better stability and improved retention in orthodontic patients.

During the winter of 1990, a distinguished group of clinicians and researchers met in Hartford, Connecticut, for a "state of the art" symposium on the stability and retention of orthodontic patients. The Connecticut temperatures were frigid—a snowstorm raged outside. There was no lack of heat in the conference hall, however, as speakers, panelists, and the audience enthusiastically considered the limitations of orthodontic stability and how improved treatment modalities can enhance short- and long-term stability. The result of their efforts is this book. A clinician will find here many sources of information to enhance his or her knowledge of stability and of methods for improving it.

We thank the contributors for their hard work and patience. We are also grateful to Raymond R. Kersey, senior editor at W. B. Saunders, and his staff for helping us with each and every step. Our special thanks to Dr. Elena-Lee Ritoli for her help during the final editing and to Dr. Andrew Kuhlberg for the cover design.

Farmington, Connecticut
March 1993

Ravindra Nanda
Charles J. Burstone

CONTENTS

PROLOGUE

Retention and Stability—
An Overview

Ravindra Nanda
and
Joseph Zernik

Every orthodontist is familiar with relapse and the need for retention. Stability of the occlusion resulting from orthodontic therapy is clearly a major goal clinicians set for themselves at the onset of treatment. Our ability to achieve long-term stability and our understanding of the factors underlying stability may be the least well founded in this triad, clear indication being our need for retention of achieved results—at times long-term retention.

Instability of the occlusion following orthodontic treatment may be divided into two general categories:

1. Changes related to growth, maturation, and aging of the dentition and the occlusion.
2. Changes related to inherent instability of the occlusion produced by orthodontic therapy.

Instability of the first type often presents over longer time periods. In this category one may include changes related to growth in preadolescent and adolescent patients—for example, deepening of the bite. Another extreme example is provided by changes related to uncoordinated growth of the maxilla and the mandible.

Changes related to maturation include increased crowding of lower incisors (Fig. 1) beyond any degree of crowding that might have been pre-

1

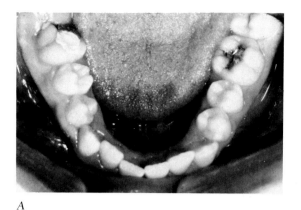

A

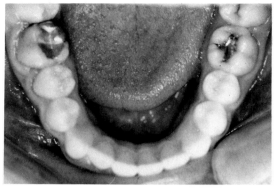

B

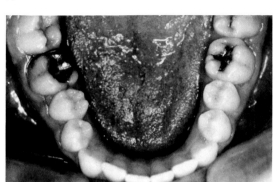

C

FIGURE 1   *A,* Lower dentition of a patient at the start of treatment. *B,* Lower arch at the end of 18 months of treatment. *C,* Lower arch three years after the end of treatment. The patient had a fixed lingual retainer from cuspid to cuspid for two years and no retainer for one year. Note that the pattern of lower incisor crowding is quite similar to pretreatment condition.

sent before treatment. Aging of the dentition is also correlated with increased incidence of periodontitis, which may be accompanied by spacing and flaring of anterior teeth, as well as by complex changes in tooth position in the semi-edentulous patient. The common theme in all of these changes is that they may very well occur in any patient, regardless of past orthodontic treatment (Fig. 2). However, the patient who is orthodontically treated expects—following the time and money invested—stability of the desired alignment achieved at the end of treatment.

These issues, analyzed in detail by Dr. Ib Leth Nielsen in Chapter 1, raise the issue of what are the effects of maxillary and mandibular growth and concomitant changes in the dentoalveolar complex on posttreatment changes and stability of treatment results. For example, Dr. Nielsen suggests that if treatment effects are directed against the specific growth direction dictated by the patient's condyles, particularly in bringing about an increase in the vertical dimension, then stability may be compromised and a relapse tendency may exist. This view is a challenge to the orthodontist who intervenes during the growth years to predict accurately the growth direction of the mandible.

Dr. Nielsen further questions the optimal treatment timing, from the stability point of view, given our knowledge of the nature of growth and development. Consistent with the view that in some cases growth may be a

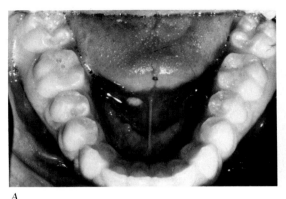
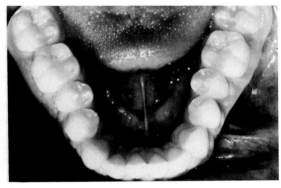

A   *B*

FIGURE 2   Lower dentition of a subject over a five-year period. No orthodontic treatment was given. *A*, Note the lower arch is almost in perfect alignment at this observation. *B*, Note the shape of the arch and the alignment of the lower incisors five years later.

major factor in determining stability, Dr. Nielsen suggests that in these patients definitive treatment, particularly extraction therapy, should be delayed until the growth pattern of the facial skeleton is clearly manifested. At a time when orthodontic treatment in the mixed dentition is gaining in popularity, this perspective is definitely unique and should be carefully studied.

Drs. Ram S. Nanda and Surender K. Nanda, in Chapter 2, join in taking the position that changes related to growth and development often influence posttreatment changes and relapse. They add detailed data, based on several of their studies, regarding changes in particular components of the craniofacial skeleton and emphasize that changes in the skeleton continue, particularly in males, well into the third decade of life.

The second category of occlusal instability involves changes that can be clearly termed as relapse and that can be directly attributed to inherent instability of the occlusion produced by orthodontic treatment. Such changes may be relatively localized, such as a bicuspid rotation that was corrected during treatment and then relapsed. The same type of rotational relapse, particularly of anterior teeth, may be a major concern to the orthodontist and the patient. Regardless of the diagnosis and treatment plan, a substantial rotation of upper central incisors can often be the initial chief complaint of a patient. Thus, relapse, even in a relatively minor and localized form, may present a substantial problem. Relapse may also involve a more generalized occlusal pattern—for example, recurrence of crowding of anterior or posterior maxillary or mandibular teeth, recurrence of crossbites, opening of extraction sites, and deepening of a corrected deep bite.

Since stability of the occlusion is a major goal of orthodontic treatment, one would expect that the orthodontist would be able to analyze and consider it in diagnosis and treatment planning. Dr. Charles Burstone, in Chapter 3, discusses numerous factors that may influence stability. Periodontal ligament and gingival fibers apparently remodel during orthodontic tooth movement. These fibers are considered responsible for some of the short-term relapse after orthodontic treatment. Particularly after rotation, the proposed solutions to this problem include overtreatment, retention, and fiberotomy. Similar mechanisms have been suggested as the basis for relapse of median maxillary diastema after orthodontic closure of the space.

Soft tissue contacts and pressure may be another major factor determining stability. The general alignment of the teeth in the alveolar bone is presumably of substantial importance. An equilibrium (Fig. 3) between the intraoral and extraoral soft tissues and function is essential for final position of teeth on alveolar bases.

To what degree are all these notions substantiated? A major dilemma in orthodontic treatment planning involves extractions in a crowded dentition. In such patients, stability of the resulting occlusion is clearly a major factor in the decision to extract. In recent years we have noticed a swinging of the pendulum toward fewer extractions. Such swings, which have apparently occurred at variable intervals in the history of orthodontics, cannot be easily explained by the appearance of dramatic new knowledge

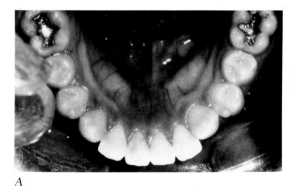

A

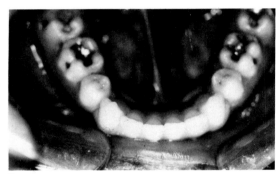

B

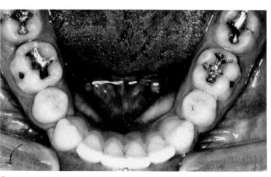

C

FIGURE 3   *A*, Lower arch of a patient at the start of treatment. Note the flared lower incisors. *B*, Lower arch at the end of treatment. Lower incisors were retracted considerably following the extraction of the first bicuspids. *C*, Lower arch five years after the end of treatment and three years after the removal of the fixed lingual cuspid-to-cuspid retainer. Note the flaring of the lower incisors.

in our field. Therefore, these swings indicate that the rationale for and pattern of our evaluation is based, at least in part, on trends and opinions voiced by unsubstantiated claims rather than on sound evidence.

Current data regarding this question are provided by Drs. Jeffrey Burzin and Ravindra Nanda in Chapter 4; John C. Gorman in Chapter 5; Robert M. Little in Chapter 6; and Cyril Sadowsky in Chapter 7.

Dr. Gorman considers stability as a goal in the context of the extraction/nonextraction debate. It is evident, he states, that extraction therapy is essential for resolving severe arch length discrepancies or protrusion. However, he raises the question whether extraction is really effective in achieving optimal incisor alignment in the long term. This question leads us directly back to examining C. H. Tweed's statement that determining the anterior limits of the denture is the key to stability. Tweed himself, however, advocated long-term fixed retention of the lower incisors in most cases. Dr. Gorman concludes that premolar extraction does not assure long-term stability of the lower incisors.

Dr. Little adds to the wealth of data generated by the ongoing studies on stability at the University of Washington, Seattle. Some of the conclusions of this long-term study may be discouraging to practitioners seeking a rational set of clear and easy to follow guidelines. According to these studies, the stability or relapse of anterior teeth following treatment cannot be predicted by any of the parameters the researchers investigated either at the onset or at the end of treatment.

Similar conclusions, derived from studies conducted at the University of Illinois, Chicago, are summarized and reported here by Dr. Sadowsky. He stresses that some degree of posttreatment relapse in the majority of patients should not be interpreted by practitioners as a license to end treatment with inferior results. Rather, these data should encourage optimal finished detailing and long-term retention.

Drs. Burzin and Nanda stress that correction of deep overbites needs careful treatment planning and that indiscriminate leveling of the occlusal plane is not the right answer from the stability standpoint. They show that the intrusion of the incisors is a viable method, from the viewpoint of stability, to correct deep overbites.

Dr. Richard G. Alexander, in Chapter 8, maintains that long-term stability is inseparable from other phases of treatment, from diagnosis and treatment planning through treatment mechanics and retention. He describes a well-formalized regimen for debanding and retention: "Countdown to Retention." This approach also includes effective and realistic patient management at this critical phase of treatment and calls for continuous retention.

Dr. Bjorn U. Zachrisson, in Chapter 9, gives numerous examples of detailed recontouring procedures, including intentional modification of tooth morphology and cosmetic procedures for long-term stability.

Dr. Arthur T. Storey, in Chapter 12, ties the question of stability to another major debate in the profession—the effect of orthodontic treat-

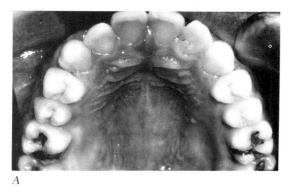

A

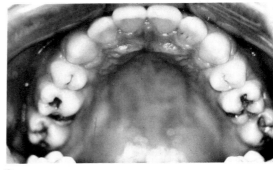

B

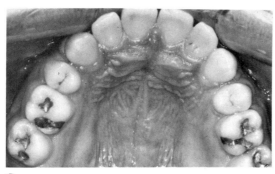

C

FIGURE 4   A, Upper arch of a patient with bimaxillary protrusion at the start of treatment. B, Patient at the end of treatment. Treatment involved extraction of the first bicuspids and retraction of the anterior teeth. C, The patient received a Hawley retainer at the end of the treatment, but never wore the retainer and did not see the orthodontist for three years. Note the flaring of the incisors, the offsetting of the extraction site, and the pattern of incisor crowding.

ment on temporomandibular joint function and dysfunction. Thus, Dr. Storey expands the definition of stability from the pure morphological criteria to include the maintenance of function. After careful examination of a variety of factors that may influence the effect of orthodontic treatment on temporomandibular joint function, he leaves the question open, calling for controlled trials to examine this point.

A similar approach is taken in Chapter 11 by Drs. Dietmar Kubein-Meesenburg and Hans Nägerl, who analyze the dentition in relation to TMJ joint function from a biomechanical point of view. This approach emphasizes that the detailed finished occlusion is a key factor in determining healthy joint function following orthodontic treatment.

Dr. Peter M. Sinclair, in Chapter 10, adds to the relapse debate the perspective of recent developments in the dynamic area of orthognathic surgery. Relapse here is primarily of surgical dentoalveolar units, and recent improvements in fixation techniques have dramatically improved the stability and predictability of surgical results.

In recent years several studies that have been initiated as clinical trials may eventually provide us with more objective data regarding the mechanisms underlying occlusal stability and the effects of treatments.

Stability of orthodontically treated dentitions is multifactorial. It starts at diagnosis and does not end at the insertion of retaining devices.

We need a long-term plan for stability. It should start at the initial consultation with patients and/or parents. The need for cooperation during and after treatment should be explained (Fig. 4). We must stress that small amounts of crowding may recur after the retaining devices are removed. Relapse should be described to the patient as a physiological event, but at the same time this fact cannot be used to hide inadequacies of diagnosis, treatment planning, and improper retaining devices (Figs. 5–8). Until we understand more about relapse and stability, it may be necessary for us to seek long-term retention with proper patient education about stability and relapse.

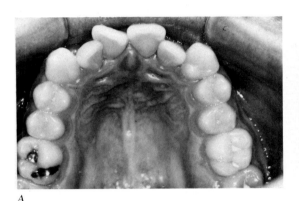
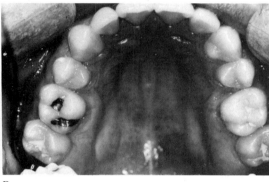

A   *B*

FIGURE 5   *A*, Upper arch of a patient prior to treatment. Note the severity of incisor crowding. *B*, Upper arch after two years of treatment and two years of Hawley retainer wear.

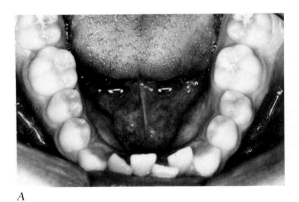
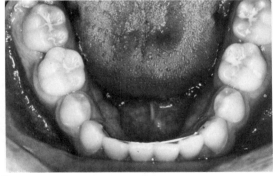

A   *B*

FIGURE 6   *A*, Lower arch of the same patient as in Figure 3 showing considerable lower crowding. *B*, Lower arch after two years of treatment and two years of retainer wear. A cuspid-to-cuspid retainer was fixed with a rigid wire retainer. Note the crowding despite the use of a retainer.

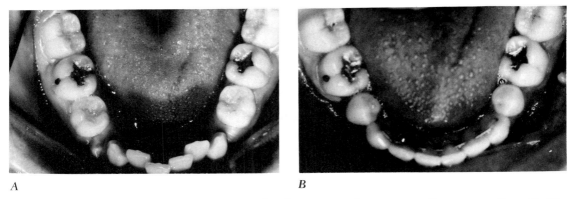

A   B

FIGURE 7   *A*, Lower arch of a patient showing significant crowding. *B*, The same patient six years after the end of treatment, still with the original fixed lingual retainer of flexible multistranded wire bonded to all the anterior teeth.

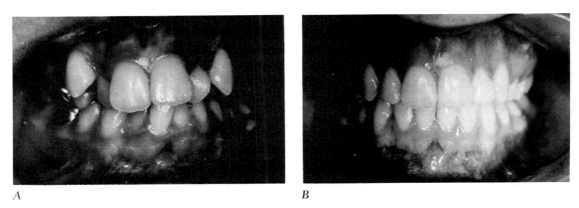

A   B

FIGURE 8   *A*, Frontal view of the anterior teeth of a patient showing crowding, overbite, and poor axial inclination of the incisors. *B*, Frontal view of the same patient six years after the end of treatment and two years after the removal of fixed lingual retainers on both upper and lower arches.

Growth Considerations in Stability of Orthodontic Treatment

Ib Leth Nielsen

INTRODUCTION

Stability of the result of orthodontic treatment has been a topic of great interest to the profession since the inception of this specialty. The problem of maintaining the teeth in their new position after treatment was recognized by Kingsley[1] in 1880, who, in a case report of a young patient with a Class II, Division 1 malocclusion, explained his concern as to the stability of retaining the teeth after treatment. Following treatment he provided the patient with a "retaining plate," but to his disappointment found, after the patient neglected to wear the retainer, that the teeth were "more disorderly than before." Based on his experience in treating various malocclusions, Kingsley further stated that "the occlusion of the teeth is the most potent factor in determining the stability in a new position"—a statement that with some modifications can be said to still hold true today.

Angle[2,3] pointed out that "as the tendency of teeth, that have been moved into occlusion, is to return to their former malposition, the main principle is the antagonizing of this force in the direction of its tendency." As to the time required to retain the treatment result, Angle offered further advice by stating that "the time of retention varies according to the age of the patient, occlusion gained, causes overcome, tooth movements accomplished, lengths of cusps, health of the tissues, etc., from a few days, to a year or two years, or often longer."

The close relationship between active orthodontic treatment and retention was emphasized by Hellman[4] who said that "retention is not a separate problem in orthodontics, but is a continuation of what we are doing during treatment." He went on to state that "we are almost completely ignorant of the specific factors causing the relapse and failures"—a statement that surprisingly still is true today.

Until the 1950s only a few studies had dealt with the problem of stability of treatment, and limited information is still available only with respect to the etiology of the lack of long-term stability. These earlier studies focused primarily on postretention changes in overjet, overbite, and intercanine and intermolar width, and on the changes in the occlusion of the teeth.

The possibility of permanently changing the dental arch width has been given particular attention in the past. Walter[5] examined the potential for changing the dental arch width and concluded that in some instances it was possible to achieve a stable result after expansion of the lower arch. Riedel[6] and Joondeph[7] in comprehensive articles discussed the various problems relating to stability following orthodontic treatment, particularly those relating to stability of the lower front teeth. Riedel[6] concluded that there was no specific pattern in which the lower incisors moved after retention. On the other hand, he observed that the maxillary incisors in 98 percent of the cases moved forward after retraction and warned against too much incisor retraction because it tended to relapse. Similar observations have been made by Rönnermann[8] and Hellekant,[9] who both reported some degree of relapse of the overjet resulting from the return of the maxillary incisors toward their original position.

The tendency for overbite, overjet and intercanine width to return toward the original was also examined by Bishara.[10] In a sample of 31 patients with four bicuspid extractions and edgewise mechanics, he studied the stability of treatment a minimum of six months out of retention. The percentage of overbite relapse was clearly greater than that of overjet relapse. He also found that the maxillary intercanine width was more stable than the mandibular intercanine width. Bishara[10] pointed out that this may be explained by the fact that "whereas the mandible continues to grow downward and forward, the maxilla is more stable" and that "the lower dentition is confined within the maxillary arch thereby assuming a smaller arch length over time."

The posttreatment stability of patients with Class I and Class II malocclusions, treated with and without extractions, was studied by Shapiro,[11] who found that Class II, Division 2 cases had a greater ability to maintain intercanine width increases in the lower arch than Class II, Division 1 and Class I cases. He further noted that the arch length reduction during treatment in the Class II, Division 2 cases was less than in the other types of malocclusions. Herberger[12] stated that all cases in his study of 56 patients 3.5 and 6 years out of retention showed some

reduction of the intercanine width in the lower arch whether they had
been treated with or without extraction therapy. On a more positive note,
Herberger[12] concluded that patients can be treated with mandibular
intercanine expansion, and in some cases a significant part of the expansion can be maintained.

In a study of 65 patients treated with first bicuspid extraction and a
minimum of 10 years out of retention, Little[13–15] found considerable individual variation in long-term response to treatment. Irrespective of Angle
classification of the initial malocclusion, amount of crowding, age, or sex,
all cases showed a decrease in arch width and arch length with time. Two
thirds of the patients had crowding in the lower arch out of retention, and
even cases that were minimally crowded before treatment showed more
crowding later. A rather discouraging finding was that the chance of maintaining lower arch alignment was less than 30 percent and that 20 percent of the cases showed marked crowding years after retention had been
discontinued.

The posttreatment changes in 72 patients treated with edgewise
mechanics, of which 27 had extractions and 45 were treated by nonextraction means, were examined by Uhde.[16] Retention of the teeth was
done with an upper Hawley appliance and a lower fixed lingual retainer.
The patients were from 12 to 35 years out of retention when the study
was performed. The findings were that overbite and overjet tended to
increase irrespective of the initial malocclusion. The molar relationships
shifted slightly toward Class II with time, and the intercuspid width was
in general unstable in the lower arch and more stable in the upper arch.
All groups showed some posttreatment crowding in the lower arch, but
less than pretreatment. No difference was found in the amount of postretention crowding between patients with extractions and those without
extractions.

Changes in overbite over time have been studied by Simons and by
Berg. Simons[17] found that patients with the deepest overbite initially, and
whose teeth were protruded during treatment, also had the deepest overbite postretention. He suggested that to enhance long-term stability
unnecessary protrusion of the mandibular anterior segment during treatment should be avoided. Berg,[18] in a follow-up study of patients 5 to 9
years out of retention, observed that of the 26 patients in the study, 24
maintained an acceptable correction long term, with a mean relapse of
the original correction of 19 percent. The tendency to relapse was slightly
greater in the Class II, Division 2 than in the Class II, Division 1 cases.
Similar observations were made by Hellekant,[9] who found no difference
between extraction and nonextraction patients in the stability of the overbite correction. He noted that cases in which the overbite remained stable
also demonstrated good stability of the intercanine width and directly
associated the changes in the lower intercanine width with the changes in
the overbite. These cases also showed the greatest amount of uprighting

of the lower incisors. The greatest change in intercanine distance was found in the extraction patients, who demonstrated a continuous decrease in this dimension

Late growth changes are among the many etiological factors that have been said to be responsible for posttreatment relapse. Riedel[19] and Moyers[20] felt that disharmonious growth following treatment may play a major role in the instability of the occlusion. That these postpubertal growth changes are common in most orthodontic patients has been shown by Björk[21] and Nanda.[22]

To improve stability several different approaches have been recommended. Of these approaches overcorrection of the posterior occlusion as well as the overbite and overjet have been the most common. Placing the lower incisors upright over basal bone, without changing the lower arch form, and treating the dental arches to a perfect intercuspidation have also been suggested as methods for reducing postretention relapse. Following treatment it has further been recommended that the teeth be retained long enough to allow bone and adjacent soft tissue to reorganize.[23,24] Extended periods of retention, in some cases until growth is terminated, and even permanent retention, have been suggested as other methods for achieving long-term stability of orthodontic results.[19]

Until now little has been done to study the association between facial growth and long-term posttreatment stability. Surprisingly few articles have dealt with the possible influence of natural growth changes on posttreatment stability. This chapter discusses the influence of maxillary and mandibular growth and the concomitant dentoalveolar development on posttreatment changes. It also considers the relationship between stability and timing of treatment, length of the subsequent retention period, and posttreatment stability.

GENERAL FACIAL GROWTH

The high variability of normal facial growth was demonstrated by Björk in 1955[25] in one of the first articles describing the use of metallic implants. In this limited study of only six patients he showed that there is great individual variation not only with respect to the direction of general facial growth, but also with respect to growth of the maxilla and mandible and to the eruption of the teeth within each jaw. Prior to the studies using implants the general feeling had been that growth was a fairly uncomplicated process and that the general direction of facial development was downward and forward, as seen in Figure 1–1. The effects of orthodontic treatment on the normal growth pattern were at that time poorly understood. An example of the influence of treatment on facial growth is seen in Figure 1–2. The superimposition shows a vertical growth pattern in a patient treated for several years with a combination of cervical headgear and a bite plate. The morphology of the mandible suggests that a more

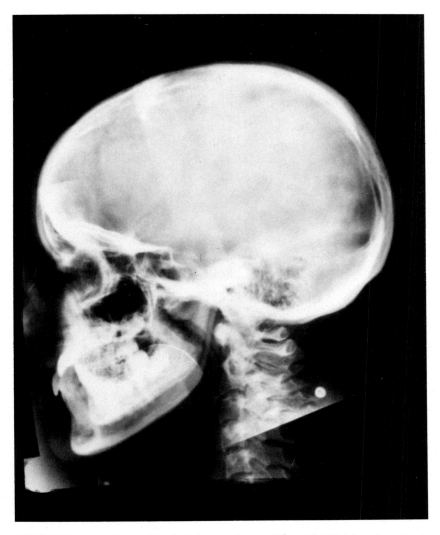

FIGURE 1–1   Favorable facial growth in a Class II, Division 1 patient between ages 7 and 14 years. The patient was treated with a functional appliance for two years and then observed for an additional five-year period.

forward-directed growth pattern was to be expected, but extrusion of the posterior teeth with the appliances has negated the favorable effects of the patient's condylar growth, resulting in vertical growth changes. Occlusal correction is possible even with this vertical growth pattern through guidance of eruption of the teeth. However, patients treated in this way finish with an unstable anterior occlusion because of the extensive dentoalveolar compensation necessary to mask the skeletal discrepancy. The teeth in such cases have a strong tendency to return to their original position.

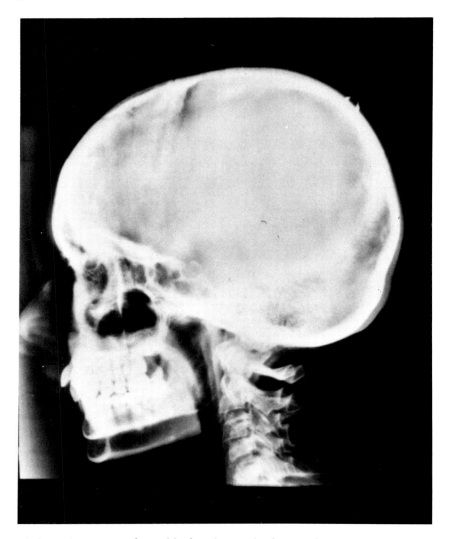

FIGURE 1–2   Unfavorable facial growth changes between ages 8 and 11 years in a young female patient treated with a Hawley bite plate and a cervical headgear. Notice that although the morphology of the mandible typically indicates a forward mandibular growth pattern, continuous extrusion of the maxillary posterior with the appliances caused the growth pattern to change.

NORMAL MANDIBULAR GROWTH

The normal growth changes of the lower jaw have been studied extensively with the use of metallic implants by Björk[25,26] and Björk and Skieller,[27,28] who examined normal mandibular growth longitudinally in a large number of subjects. Their studies of patients, using metallic implants, showed great individual variation in the growth pattern of the lower jaw. With the aid of metallic implants placed within the jaw bones the actual growth changes can be more accurately demonstrated, without the influence of surface modeling that with conventional analysis techniques masks the actual growth changes. This modeling on average disguises as much as 50 percent of the growth rotations of the lower jaw.[27] If this is not taken into consideration in evaluating growth and dentoalveolar changes, it can lead to incorrect interpretations, as demonstrated by Isaacson.[29]

In a detailed study of mandibular growth Björk[21] showed that the range of variation of condylar growth in untreated normal subjects may be as much as 42° with a slight upward and forward growth direction being the most common. In his sample of 25 boys, Björk[21] found that while some subjects showed the condyles to grow upward and forward, others showed an almost posterior growth direction. Associated with this variability in condylar growth were distinct variations in the direction of eruption of teeth.

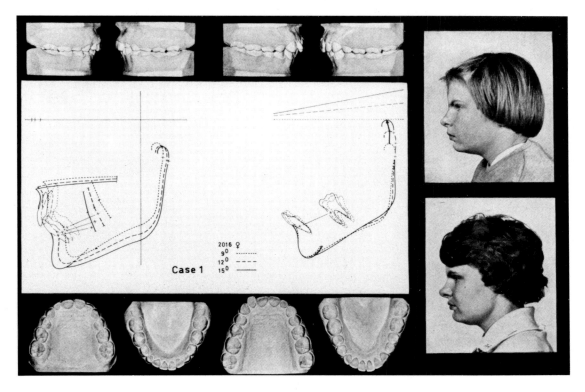

FIGURE 1–3 Facial growth and occlusal development in an untreated subject with pronounced forward rotation of the mandible. Notice the occlusion has remained stable during this six-year growth period without any crowding developing in the lower arch. (From Björk A, Skieller V: Facial development and tooth eruption. Am J Orthod 62:339, 1972.)

In most subjects with pronounced forward condylar growth, the lower posterior teeth erupt and migrate mesially (Figs. 1–3 and 1–4). If, however, the lower incisors are prevented from moving forward—for example, by a deep bite—increased crowding in the lower arch often develops. In cases where the tendency to mesial migration is pronounced, it is therefore not surprising that the intercanine width in the lower arch also tends to decrease because the teeth move into a more narrow part of the arch. The degree to which this "secondary crowding" develops is dependent upon several local factors, such as the extent of overbite, overjet, available space in the arch, and inclination of the maxillary and mandibular anterior front teeth, as well as the extent of mesial migration of the posterior teeth.

Patients with upward-backward growth of the condyles, in contrast, consistently show a more vertical direction of eruption of the posterior teeth (Figs. 1–5 and 1–6). However, these patients also develop secondary

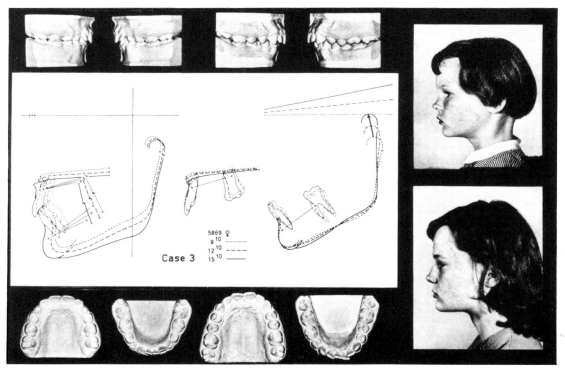

FIGURE 1–4 Facial growth and occlusal development in an untreated subject with pronounced forward mandibular growth rotation and a stable anterior occlusion. The growth pattern in this subject is similar to that of the patient seen in Figure 1–3. This subject developed crowding of the mandibular incisors with time. Notice the posterior occlusion change from an end-on relationship at age 9 years, 10 months to a full Class II malocclusion at age 15 years, 10 months. (From Björk A, Skieller V: Facial development and tooth eruption. Am J Orthod 62:339, 1972.)

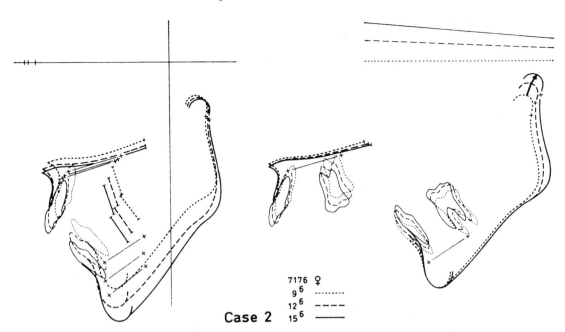

FIGURE 1–5   Facial growth in an untreated subject with an anterior open bite and pronounced posterior growth of the mandibular condyles. Notice the uprighting of the mandibular molars and incisors during this six-year growth period. (From Björk A, Skieller V: Facial development and tooth eruption. Am J Orthod 62:339, 1972.)

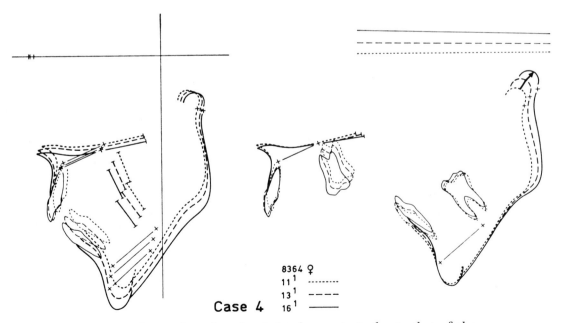

FIGURE 1–6   Facial growth and occlusal development similar to that of the patient in Figure 1–5. Notice the almost identical uprighting of the lower incisors but with much less eruption of the molars. (From Björk A, Skieller V: Facial development and tooth eruption. Am J Orthod 62:339, 1972.)

crowding as the lower incisors erupt in a more posterior direction, uprighting on the jaw base. The extent of uprighting of the incisors is influenced and modified by the balance between the lower lip and the tongue, by the space conditions in the arch, and by the growth changes of the mandible.

STABILITY OF OCCLUSION AND MANDIBULAR GROWTH ROTATION

ANTERIOR ROTATION

Rotational growth changes of the lower jaw were first described by Björk in 1969.[30] He reported that pronounced upward-forward growth of the mandibular condyles is associated with anterior or counterclockwise rotation of the lower jaw. This rotation can occur with a fulcrum point located at the incisors or further back in the occlusion. When the occlusion remains stable over time, the fulcrum point is located and maintained at the incisors, presumably by the function of the lips and tongue. However, if the fulcrum point is lost, as a result of dysfunction of the lips or tongue or because of oral habits, a skeletal deep bite will normally develop (Fig. 1–7). The rotational growth changes in normal subjects are the result of a greater increase in posterior face height (PFH) than in anterior face height (AFH).[31] In patients in which anterior rotation is to be expected *the goal of orthodontic treatment is to establish and maintain normal overbite and overjet relationships by creating a solid fulcrum point at the incisors.* By positioning the teeth so that the interincisal angle is not too obtuse, the lower incisors are not too upright, and there is a proper amount of torque of the maxillary incisors, a more stable result can be anticipated. In other words, the concept that the lower incisors must be placed at right angles to the mandibular plane, as proposed by Tweed,[32] is not the answer to obtaining long-term stability in cases with pronounced anterior rotation. The normal uprighting tendency of the incisors will, as they follow the jaw rotation, result in loss of the fulcrum point with deepening of the bite and increased crowding of the mandibular anterior teeth. More important, therefore, than positioning the lower teeth at a certain angle to the lower jaw may be how these teeth are placed relative to the upper teeth and to the soft tissue matrix, while at the same time taking into consideration the bony support and the periodontal tissues.

In addition to creating an optimal anterior and posterior occlusion, at the end of active treatment it is also necessary to maintain and support this occlusion with retention appliances. In extreme cases retention must be continued until growth of the condyles is completed because following active treatment there is often an even greater tendency toward anterior rotation than during treatment.

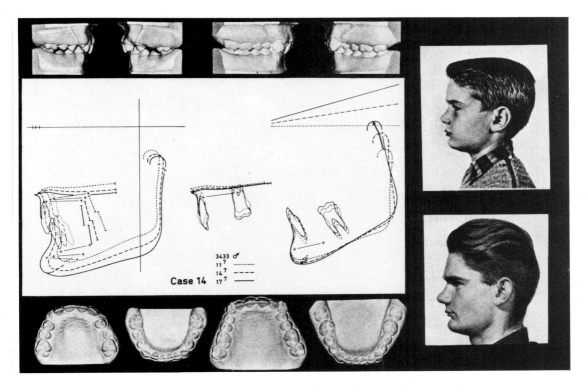

Case 14

FIGURE 1–7   Facial growth and occlusal development in a subject with an extreme deep bite. The lack of a fulcrum point at the incisors in combination with the growth pattern has resulted in continuous deepening of the bite. The general superimposition shows that the mandibular molars continued to upright while the maxillary molars became more mesially inclined over time. The maxilla in this patient rotated forward, similar to the mandible. Notice the increasing crowding in the maxillary arch resulting from mesial migration of the posterior teeth and retroclination of the anterior teeth. This occlusal development is characteristic of the Class II, Division 2 malocclusion.

Patients with severe malocclusions, for example, Class II skeletal malocclusions and a deep bite, where early treatment may be indicated and who have a more extreme growth pattern, present additional stability problems. In these cases the mandibular anterior teeth must be maintained in their new position for a long time because the continuing forward-growth rotation usually is accompanied by uprighting of the teeth. Stabilizing the lower incisors presents a practical problem, however, because the stability of the anterior mandible is compromised when the primary canines are lost. A fixed lingual retainer, banded to the second primary or first permanent molars, in combination with a passive bite plate that does not take the posterior teeth out of occlusion, can often prevent the deep bite from returning. A functional appliance worn at night throughout this period may similarly help prevent relapse of the original malocclusion by supporting the anterior occlusion.

When the permanent mandibular canines are fully erupted in the late mixed dentition, retention is often simpler. The canines can then aid in supporting the lower anterior teeth against the uprighting tendency of the mandibular incisors. At this stage an upper Hawley retainer provided with a bite plane will assist in preventing the lower incisors from overerupting and is used in combination with a lower fixed lingual 3×3 or 4×4 retainer.

POSTERIOR ROTATION

In patients with upward-backward condylar growth, the amount of effective vertical condylar growth, which primarily determines PFH increase, is often minimal. As the increase in AFH in these subjects normally exceeds the increase in PFH, the result is backward or posterior rotation of the mandible.[31] This type of growth rotation is, however, much less common than anterior rotation seen in the majority of our patients during growth. Because the direction of eruption of the lower incisors is more vertical, with additional potential for retroclination of these teeth, there is a strong tendency toward late lower crowding. Therefore, long-term stabilization of the lower anterior teeth is absolutely necessary.

MAXILLARY GROWTH AND STABILITY

Growth of the maxilla has been shown to be associated with rotations similar to those observed in the mandible.[33] In untreated subjects these rotational changes are normally in the same direction as in the lower jaw but of less intensity. Concomitant with the rotation of the maxilla is the continuous mesial migration of the upper posterior teeth similar to that seen in the mandible. In the maxilla, as in the mandible, there is often less forward movement of the anterior than of the posterior teeth, resulting in gradually increasing anterior crowding. As in the development of lower crowding, the function of the lips may also play an important role in the development of maxillary anterior crowding. It may be hypothesized that the lips are preventing the upper front teeth from following the mesial migration of the posterior teeth. A recent study by Thüer,[34] however, showed that the upper lip in Class II, Division 2 cases is either hypotonic or has normal activity. It is possible that the lower lip might be an important etiologic factor in the development of upper crowding. Another possibility is that normal lip function, in combination with a more extreme tendency toward anterior rotation of the maxilla, may be sufficient to redirect the eruption of the incisors. The same mechanisms may be responsible for the posttreatment relapse of maxillary anterior crowding. This occlusal development is particularly characteristic of the Class II, Division 2 malocclusions, where the upper anterior teeth usually show increased crowding with time (Fig. 1–7). Note the increased crowding in the maxilla at age 17 years, 7 months. The lower arch shows no crowding despite the lack of forward movement of the incisors in combination with some mesial migration of the posterior teeth. This can in part be attributed to some existing space at age 11 years, 7 months and in part to a broadening of the arch form over time.

In subjects with more pronounced forward-growth rotation of the jaws, there is a natural tendency for the molar relationship to become more Class II with time, as observed by Uhde.[16] This can also be attributed to the natural growth changes, where the posterior teeth in both arches tend to follow the growth rotations of the jaws, and therefore become more mesially inclined in the maxilla and more distally inclined or upright in the mandible.[27] Because molars shift in opposite directions, the occlusion gradually shifts toward a Class II malocclusion. These changes can be more or less pronounced, depending on the intercuspidation and the function of the soft tissue matrix.[35]

DYSPLASTIC AND COMPENSATORY DEVELOPMENT

Skeletal discrepancies are often to a great extent masked by dentoalveolar compensation.[35] In some subjects, however, abnormal function of the lips and tongue can cause dysplastic dentoalveolar changes that make the dental malocclusion worse than the underlying skeletal problem. The extent of compensation not only influences the occlusal correction necessary to treat the case but also affects posttreatment stability. Just as compensatory and dysplastic development is greatly dependent upon the soft tissue matrix surrounding the skeleton, posttreatment stability is dependent upon the adaptability of these structures. Our knowledge of the influence of functional factors on occlusal development is unfortunately still rather limited, and only a few studies have addressed these problems.[36,37]

DENTOALVEOLAR DEVELOPMENT AND OCCLUSION

The continuous forward movement of the posterior teeth in patients with forward rotation of the mandible is necessary to maintain stability of the anterior occlusion. Anteriorly this migration is reflected primarily as proclination of the lower incisors, as seen in Figures 1–3 and 1–4. These two patients are from a sample of 21 cases with metallic implants, where facial growth was studied during a six-year period around puberty by Björk and Skieller.[27] Both subjects maintained a stable anterior occlusion despite pronounced forward mandibular growth rotation. The interincisal angle in both instances remained constant during the growth period, and only minimal changes in the overbite and overjet took place. Both subjects experienced a similar amount of forward-growth rotation of the lower jaw, as seen by the change in the inclination of the nasion-sella lines on the mandibular superimposition. In one case (Case 3, Fig. 1–4) increased crowding of the mandibular incisors developed, whereas the other subject (Case 1, Fig. 1–3) showed no change in the space conditions. These two cases demonstrate why the goal of orthodontic treatment in this type of growth pattern should be to bring the mandibular dentition forward on the jaw base and maintain the anterior teeth in their forward position so as to counteract the natural tendency of the incisors to upright.

STABILITY OF EXTRACTION AND NONEXTRACTION TREATMENT

In the patient with a growth pattern in which there is a pronounced tendency toward anterior rotation, extractions, especially of teeth in the lower arch, should normally be avoided. The potential for sagittal and transverse expansion must be carefully examined before any decision is made to remove bicuspids. In the past the policy has too often been to focus primarily on the amount of crowding and on the inclination of the lower mandibular anterior teeth without giving consideration to facial growth pattern and rotational growth changes of the jaws. As a result, treatment has often been finished with an unstable occlusion, with the lower front teeth too upright, accompanied by an obtuse interincisal angle that lacks an anterior fulcrum point.

When extractions are necessary to alleviate crowding, they should not be carried out too early but rather during the growth spurt or even later when the growth pattern in the patient is more clearly expressed. Following treatment, retention is even more critical in these extraction cases because the lower incisors often are more upright at the end of treatment than in nonextraction cases and therefore must be maintained until growth of the condyles is completed.

Where condylar growth is primarily directed posteriorly, the natural tendency of the mandibular incisors to become more crowded with time continues throughout the growth period. It is therefore critical that extraction decisions not be made too early. In fact, *in most instances where posterior rotation is anticipated, extractions should be delayed until the patient is past maximum pubertal growth.* The degree of growth rotation and associated natural tooth migration in these cases is unpredictable, and additional late crowding, resulting from the growth pattern, will often develop even after extraction therapy. Following treatment, the mandibular anterior teeth in these patients should be supported lingually until growth in the mandible is finished. Two examples of this growth pattern are seen in Figures 1–5 and 1–6. Note the tooth movements in the lower arch where the mandibular superimposition shows that the posterior teeth in both subjects erupt almost vertically, while the anterior teeth upright.

Both patients developed increasing crowding of the anterior teeth. The change in the inclination of the nasion-sella line, seen on the mandibular superimposition, reflects the degree of posterior rotation during this six-year period of growth without treatment.

TREATMENT TIMING

The majority of orthodontic treatments are carried out immediately prior to or during the pubertal growth spurt. In some instances, however, treatment during the early mixed dentition stage may be indicated. One reason early treatment has come into some discredit is that these cases are often associated with even greater instability posttreatment than when treatment is done in the late mixed or permanent dentition stage. The lack of supporting teeth posteriorly in the arch, when the deciduous teeth are lost, increases the chances for uprighting of the anterior teeth, resulting in a deep bite. The mandibular anterior teeth, therefore, need to be supported until the permanent canines are fully erupted. The need for a long retention period to maintain the correction has often been ignored by clinicians, who in early treatment cases often have either no retention period or discontinue retention too soon. This has brought early treatment into some discredit as a means of intercepting the developing malocclusion

The majority of malocclusions are primarily related to skeletal differences between the maxilla and mandible, and the goal of treatment is to correct this discrepancy by so-called growth adaptation. One of the primary objectives of treatment in Class II patients, for example, is to take maximum advantage of forward growth of the mandible while restraining maxillary forward growth in some way. To obtain maximum effect, treatment is often carried out during the pubertal growth period, when the intensity of growth is at its greatest. Whereas facial growth can be of great help during treatment of a skeletal problem, it can also be the cause of instability of the treatment result. As growth in most orthodontic patients is not completed at the end of the growth spurt but continues for several years beyond the pubertal spurt, retention of the treatment result should also continue for a period of several years.

Growth of the mandible, after having reached a peak at $14^1/_2$ years on average in males, slows down in intensity until completion, which on average occurs at age 19 years (Fig. 1–8). The graph, based on a sample of 25 Scandinavian boys,[21] also illustrates that the range of variation for completion of growth of the mandible is as much as 8 years, with the earliest completion seen at age 15 and the latest at age 23 years. This demonstrates the necessity for long-term retention, especially of the lower arch, in cases where residual growth is a critical factor with respect to long-term stability. In these patients retention may, in the extreme case, have to be maintained until the age of 22 to 23 years. Figure 1–8 further shows that maxillary growth on average is completed 2 to $2^1/_2$ years prior

cm/mm per year

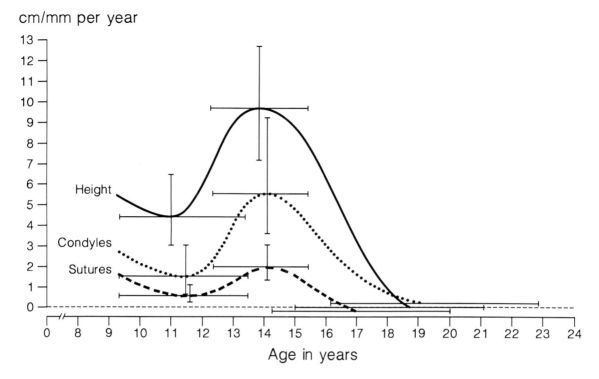

FIGURE 1–8   Mean annual growth rates and individual variations in body height, condyles, and sutures in boys. The pubertal maximum in height is seen at age 14 years. Completion of sutural growth occurs on average at age 17 years and of condylar growth at age 19 years. Notice the large range of variation. (Redrawn from Björk A: Sutural growth of the upper face studied by the implant method. Acta Odontol Scand 24:109, 1966.)

to mandibular growth. The timepoint for completion of sutural growth again varies by as much as 6 years, with the earliest completion of maxillary growth at age 14 years and the latest at age 20 years. This differential in timing, between completion of upper and lower jaw growth, is yet another factor that influences posttreatment stability. If we further consider that in individual cases it is not uncommon for growth of the maxillary sutures to be completed at the early end of this range and for mandibular growth to be completed late, the potential for considerable changes in the sagittal maxillo-mandibular relationship develops. It is not surprising under these circumstances, therefore, that the dentoalveolar structures may have difficulty in masking the discrepancies, resulting in crowding and relapse of the orthodontic overbite-overjet correction. In order to illustrate the integration of potential growth rotations into the diagnosis, treatment, and retention planning the following selected case is presented.

CASE D. H., MALE, AGE 12 YEARS, 9 MONTHS
(Figs. 1–9 through 1–13)

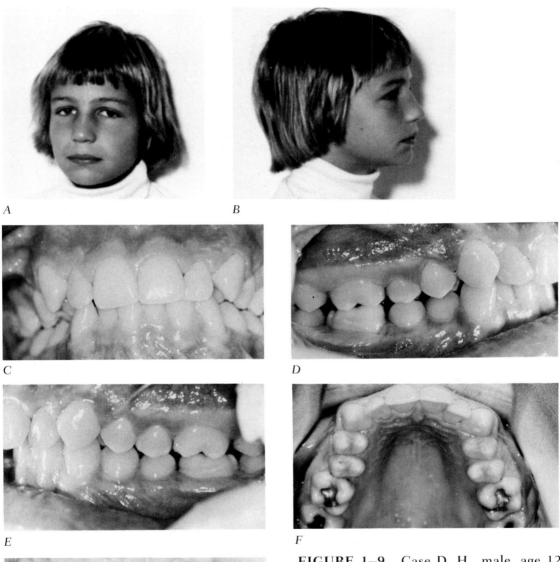

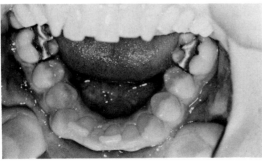

FIGURE 1–9 Case D. H., male, age 12 years, 9 months. *A* and *B*, Facial photo shows a moderately retrognathic mandible. Lip closure is adequate, and there is no lip strain. *C* to *G*, Intraoral photos show a Class II, Division 2 malocclusion with a deep bite. There is a buccal crossbite on the left side. The maxillary dental arch shows a moderate amount of crowding. The mandibular arch shows pronounced crowding and a constricted dental arch in the bicuspid region.

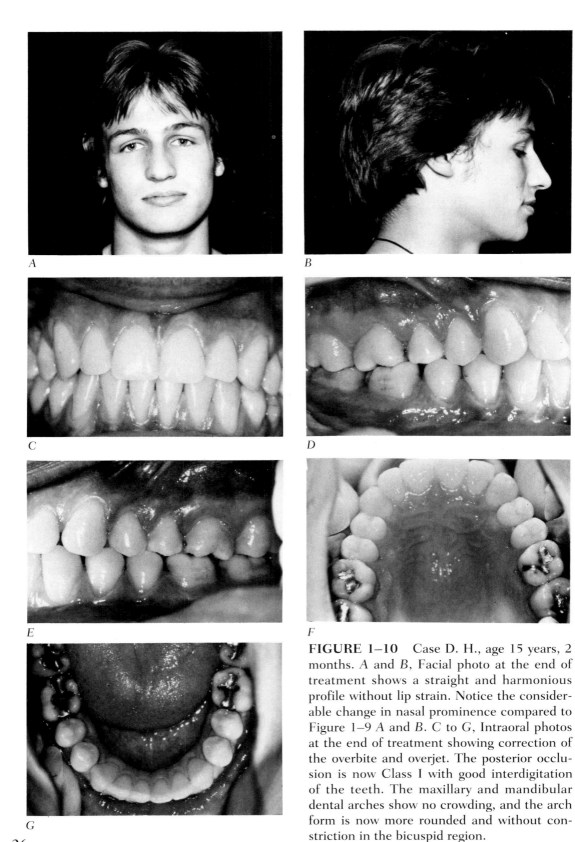

FIGURE 1–10 Case D. H., age 15 years, 2 months. *A* and *B*, Facial photo at the end of treatment shows a straight and harmonious profile without lip strain. Notice the considerable change in nasal prominence compared to Figure 1–9 *A* and *B*. *C* to *G*, Intraoral photos at the end of treatment showing correction of the overbite and overjet. The posterior occlusion is now Class I with good interdigitation of the teeth. The maxillary and mandibular dental arches show no crowding, and the arch form is now more rounded and without constriction in the bicuspid region.

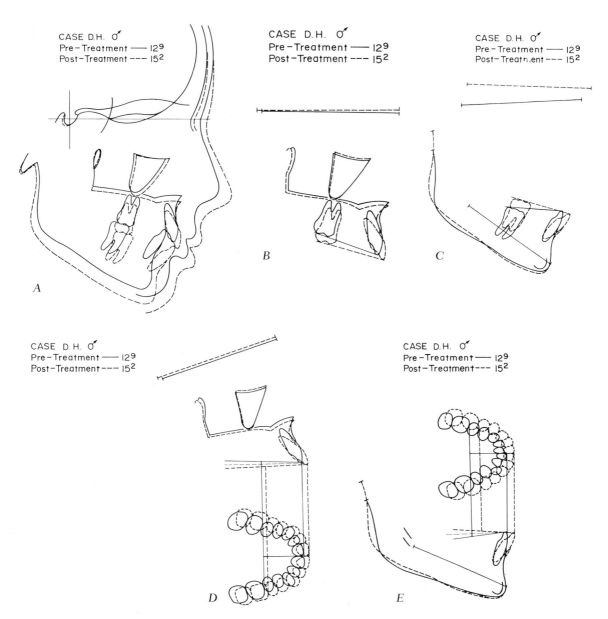

FIGURE 1–11 Case D. H. *A,* Cephalometric growth and treatment analysis of the treatment period show that facial growth in general had been downward and forward. Maxilla growth was primarily vertical, whereas the mandible grew downward and forward. *B,* Maxillary superimposition shows that the maxilla rotated slightly posteriorly during treatment. The maxillary incisors were torqued to obtain good occlusion with the mandibular incisors. *C,* Mandibular superimposition shows uprighting of the mandibular incisors and moderate eruption of the lower molars. Notice the pronounced forward rotation during this period, as seen by the change in the inclination of the nasion sella lines. *D,* The maxillary dental arch had been widened during treatment, about 3 mm over the first molars. *E,* The mandibular arch was expanded about 6 mm in the area of the first molars and 9 mm in the region of the bicuspids. In the cuspid region the expansion was only 1.5 mm.

The patient has a Class II, Division 2 malocclusion and a deep bite. There is a 2-mm midline deviation to the right of the mandibular teeth and a buccal crossbite on the right side. The mandibular crowding is estimated at 6 mm and the upper arch crowding at about 5 mm.

The Class II malocclusion is skeletal and is due to an increased sagittal jaw relation (ss-n-pg) (5° ≈ mean 2°) primarily associated with a retrognathic mandible (75° ≈ mean 80°). The maxilla is also slightly retrognathic (80° ≈ mean 82°). The maxillary incisors are compensatorily retroclined, but the dentoalveolar compensation does not adequately mask the skeletal discrepancy.

The deep bite is dentoalveolar and the result of the previous growth pattern and overeruption of both the upper and lower incisors. The transverse malocclusion is primarily dentoalveolar and the result of lingual tipping of the lower bicuspids in addition to some narrowing of the upper arch in the bicuspid region.

Based on the morphology of the mandible and the structural signs, as described by Björk,[30] it was anticipated that the patient would have a significant amount of anterior or forward rotation of the lower jaw with a downward and forward growth pattern during his residual growth period. A hand-wrist plate taken at this time showed the patient to be about one to two years prior to puberty, indicating that a significant amount of growth could be expected in the following two to three years. The amount of crowding, together with the fact that the lower arch showed lingual inclination of the bicuspids, suggested that it would be possible to expand both the lower arch and the similarly narrow upper arch. In addition, it was felt that the growth pattern, in particular the potential for mandibular forward rotation, further indicated that treatment could be carried out without extractions because the lower dental arch can normally be brought forward on the base to create a fulcrum point at the incisors, as indicated previously. The treatment goals were to (1) alleviate the crowding by expansion of both arches, (2) correct the Class II malocclusion by growth adaptation, (3) correct the midline discrepancy by tooth movement, and (4) reduce the deep bite by a combination of intrusion of the anterior teeth in both jaws and eruption of the posterior teeth.

Treatment was initiated by expanding the lower arch with a quad-Helix appliance. This was followed by more moderate expansion of the upper arch in a similar way. The Class II correction was accomplished in part by the use of a cervical headgear and in part by Class II elastics. The Class II elastics were used to intentionally bring the lower arch forward on the jaw base. In other words, in this patient Class II elastics assisted in sustaining the normal mesial migration of the teeth and also helped correct the Class II molar relationship.

After 2 years, 5 months of treatment the treatment goals were achieved and the appliances were removed. The facial photo at this time shows a straight profile with a slightly prominent nose. The occlusion is now Class I, with normal overbite and overjet, and all crowding has been eliminated.

To retain the occlusion a lower 4 × 4 retainer was inserted. In the upper arch a Hawley retainer with a flat bite plane was placed, which allowed the posterior teeth to remain in occlusion. A 4 × 4 retainer was preferred in this patient because of the expansion of the lower arch during treatment. The bite plane on the upper Hawley retainer was intended to prevent the lower incisors from overerupting into a deep bite, in case the teeth were able to further erupt in spite of the 4 × 4 retainer.

The patient was asked to wear the upper retainer at all times except during meals for the first three months and thereafter at night only. Retention was maintained for 2 years, 5 months, until the patient was past puberty and a hand-wrist plate showed completion of growth in all epiphyses.

Analysis of the cephalometric headfilm, taken at the end of active treatment, shows that the general facial growth direction had been downward and forward. The superimpositions in Figure 1–11A made on the anterior cranial base structures, as described by Björk[28] demonstrate that growth of the maxilla had been primarily vertical, whereas the mandible had grown downward and forward. This growth direction had helped correct the Class II malocclusion and improve the relationship of the mandible to the maxilla. The maxillary molars had been held back by the headgear, while the mandibular molars had been carried forward by the growth of the mandible, correcting the malocclusion. Superimposition of the maxilla on the anterior outline of the zygomatic process[38] shows that the upper incisors were torqued considerably to obtain a good interincisal angle, thereby securing the fulcrum point. There was a slight posterior rotation of the maxilla during the treatment period, as seen in the change of the nasion-sella line. Mandibular structural superimposition[30] (Fig. 1–11C) shows considerable proclination of the lower incisors with mesial movement of the lower molars. In spite of pronounced eruption of the lower posterior teeth, some forward growth rotation of the lower jaw took place during treatment. This can be ascribed to the amount of condylar growth that this patient experienced during the 2 years and 5 months of treatment that exceeded the eruption of the teeth.

Maxillary and mandibular superimpositions, including the occlusograms (Figs. 1–11D and E), show that both arches were expanded considerably during treatment. In fact, the expansion of the mandibular arch was as much as 6 mm measured at the first molars and 9 mm at the bicuspids, whereas in the mandibular canine region the expansion was only 1.5 mm. The expansion in the maxillary molar and bicuspid regions was about half as much.

The photos of the study casts 2 years, 6 months out of retention show a stable occlusion with a normal overbite and overjet. The third molars have now also erupted into occlusion. Both the upper and lower

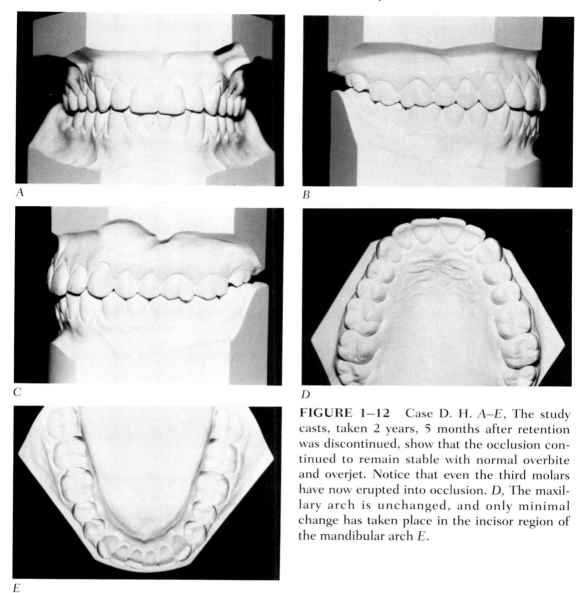

FIGURE 1–12 Case D. H. A–E, The study casts, taken 2 years, 5 months after retention was discontinued, show that the occlusion continued to remain stable with normal overbite and overjet. Notice that even the third molars have now erupted into occlusion. D, The maxillary arch is unchanged, and only minimal change has taken place in the incisor region of the mandibular arch E.

dental arches remained virtually unchanged, and only minimal change is seen in the lower incisor position. Cephalometric analysis, out of retention, shows that a considerable amount of growth took place during the period from the end of treatment to out of retention (Fig. 1–13A). During this period mandibular growth was even more anteriorly directed than during active treatment. The maxillary growth direction changed from vertical to downward-forward following that of the mandible. This change may be ascribed to the fact that no orthodontic/orthopedic forces affected the maxilla directly during the posttreatment period. The pronounced for-

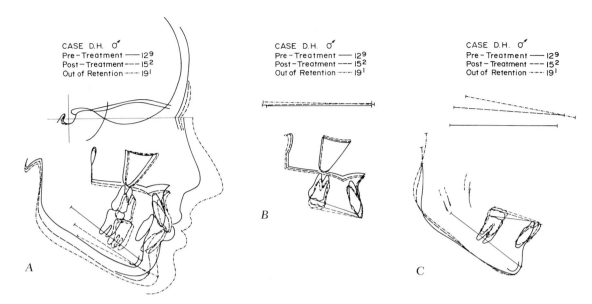

FIGURE 1–13   Case D. H. *A,* Cephalometric growth and treatment analysis, 2 years, 6 months out of retention, show that general facial growth continued in a downward-forward direction. However, maxillary growth is now more forwardly directed than during treatment. Notice the uprighting of the mandibular incisors relative to the profile. *B,* Maxillary superimposition shows no change in maxillary incisor position, whereas the molars continued to erupt moderately. *C,* Mandibular superimposition shows uprighting of the mandibular incisors and very little eruption of the molars. The forward growth rotation during this period was pronounced as a result of continued condylar growth and very limited eruption of the molars.

ward rotation of the mandible during this period was associated with moderate uprighting of the lower incisors relative to the face.

Maxillary superimposition (Fig. 1–13*B*) shows a slight forward rotation of the maxilla during the second period, in contrast to the posterior rotation seen during treatment. This change may be attributed to the discontinuation of orthodontic forces to the maxilla.

Mandibular superimposition shows pronounced forward-growth rotation during the posttreatment period (Fig. 1–13*C*). The lower incisors uprighted on the mandible in part as a result of the removal of the lower 4 × 4 retainer and in part as a result of the uprighting that occurred through the forward-growth rotation of the mandible. Eruption of the mandibular molars during this period was moderate compared to the eruption seen during treatment. This difference again may be attributed to treatment effects from the arch wires and the Class II elastics.

In general when this patient's posttreatment facial profile is considered, it was fortunate extractions were not undertaken in this case. With the amount of growth of the nose in this patient, extraction of four bicuspids with subsequent retraction of the anterior teeth would have left the individual with a very undesirable profile. In addition, it is seen from the superimpositions that proclination of the lower incisors in this growth pattern was desirable to create a stable anterior occlusion, which then had to be maintained during the posttreatment period during which growth continued for several years. Extraction therapy in this growth pattern would have made establishing a fulcrum point difficult, and the bite would most likely have collapsed, resulting not only in lower arch crowding but also in a recurrence of the deep bite.

SUMMARY

This chapter discussed the role of facial growth as an etiological factor in the long-term instability of orthodontic treatment often reported in the literature. The focus has primarily been on facial growth and dentoalveolar development. However, the dentoalveolar changes described here are not only the result of the influence of growth on tooth movement but also a function of the soft tissue matrix surrounding the hard tissue structures. Unfortunately, our knowledge about the role of the soft tissues in the development of malocclusion and the ability of these tissues to adapt to the changes accomplished through treatment is still limited, and further research in this area is greatly needed.

Many of the postretention changes, such as crowding of the mandibular and maxillary incisors, relapse of the overbite and overjet, and return toward a previous Class II occlusion can be explained as being primarily due to posttreatment growth changes. However, other long-term changes such as relapse of a single rotated tooth or an anterior open bite, spacing of the teeth, and so on, may be explained as primarily due to more local factors, including inability of the periodontal fibers to reorganize, compromised airways, and lack of adaptability of the soft tissues.

There is little doubt, however, that growth—in particular, residual growth—influences the posttreatment stability of orthodontic treatment. Not enough attention has been given to this aspect of orthodontic diagnosis and treatment planning. The dynamics of facial development and the normal variations in maxillary and mandibular growth, with the concomitant dentoalveolar development, need to be better understood before we can expect to create more stable treatment results. To enhance long-term stability, the anticipated facial growth changes in a patient should always be considered and should be included in the planning not only of the active orthodontic treatment but of the retention period after treatment.

REFERENCES

1. Kingsley NW: Oral Deformities. New York, D. Appleton and Company, 1880, p. 136.
2. Angle EH: Retention. *In* Angle EH (ed.): Treatment of Malocclusion of the Teeth. Philadelphia, PA, S. S. White Dental Manufacturing Company, 1907, pp. 263–304.
3. Angle EH: Retention. *In* Angle EH (ed.): Treatment of Malocclusion of the Teeth and Fractures of the Maxillae. Philadelphia, PA, S. S. White Dental Manufacturing Company, 1900, Chapter XII.
4. Hellman M: Fundamental principles and expedient promises in orthodontic procedures. *In* Transactions of the American Association of Orthodontists. St. Louis, MO, C. V. Mosby, 1945, p. 46.
5. Walter DC: Changes in the form and dimensions of dental arches resulting from orthodontic treatment. Angle Orthod 23:3–18, 1953.
6. Riedel RA: A review of the retention problem. Angle Orthod 30:179–199, 1960.
7. Joondeph DR, Riedel RA: "Retention." *In* Graber TM, Swain BF (eds.): Orthodontics: Current Orthodontic Principles and Techniques. St. Louis, MO, C. V. Mosby, 1985.
8. Rönnerman A, Larsson E: Overjet, overbite, intercanine distance and root resorption in orthodontically treated patients. Swed Dent J 5:21–27, 1981.
9. Hellekant M, Lagerström L, Gleerup A: Overbite and overjet correction in a Class II, Division 1 sample treated with Edgewise therapy. Eur J Orthod 11:91–106, 1989.
10. Bishara SE, Chadha JM, Potter RB: Stability of intercanine width, overbite and overjet correction. Am J Orthod 63:588–595, 1963.
11. Shapiro PA: Mandibular dental arch form and dimension. Treatment and posttreatment changes. Am J Orthod 66:58–70, 1974.
12. Herberger RJ: Stability of mandibular intercuspid width after long periods of retention. Angle Orthod 51:78–83, 1981.
13. Little RM, Wallen TR, Riedel RA: Stability and relapse of mandibular anterior alignment—first premolar extraction cases treated by traditional edgewise orthodontics. Am J Orthod 80:349–365, 1981.
14. Little MR, Riedel RA: Postretention evaluation of stability and relapse—Mandibular arches with generalized spacing. Am J Orthod Dentofacial Orthop 95:37–41, 1989.
15. Little R, Riedel R, Årtun J: An evaluation of changes in mandibular anterior alignment from 10 to 20 years postretention. Am J Orthod 93:423–428, 1988.
16. Uhde MD, Sadowsky C, BeGole EA: Long-term stability of dental relationships after orthodontic treatment. Angle Orthod 53:240–252, 1983.
17. Simons ME, Joondeph DR: Change in overbite: A ten-year postretention study. Am J Orthod 64:349–367, 1973.
18. Berg R: Stability of overbite correction. Eur J Orthod 5:75–83, 1983.
19. Riedel RA: Retention. *In* Graber TM, Swain BF (eds.): Current Orthodontic Concepts and Techniques, 2nd. ed. Philadelphia, PA, W. B. Saunders, 1975.
20. Moyers RE: Handbook of Orthodontics, 4th ed. Chicago, Year Book Publishers, Inc., 1988, pp. 326–327.

21. Björk A: Sutural growth of the upper face studied by the implant method. Acta Odontol Scand 24:109–127, 1966.
22. Nanda RS: The rates of growth of several facial components measured from serial cephalometric roentgenograms. Am J Orthod 41:658–673, 1955.
23. Reitan K: Principles of retention and avoidance of posttreatment relapse. Am J Orthod 55:776–790, 1969.
24. Reitan K: Clinical and histological observations on tooth movement during and after orthodontic treatment. Am J Orthod 53:721–745, 1967.
25. Björk A: Facial growth in man studied with the aid of metallic implants. Acta Odontol Scand 13:9–34, 1955.
26. Björk A: Variations in the growth pattern of the human mandible: Longitudinal radiographic study by the implant method. J Dent Res 42:400–411, 1963.
27. Björk A, Skieller V: Facial development and tooth eruption. Am J Orthod 62:339–383, 1972.
28. Björk A, Skieller V: Normal and abnormal growth of the mandible: A synthesis of longitudinal cephalometric implant studies over a period of 25 years. Eur J Orthod 5:1–46, 1983.
29. Isaacson RJ, Worms FW, Speidel TM: Measurement of tooth movement. Amer J Orthod 70:290–303, 1976.
30. Björk A: Prediction of mandibular growth rotation. Am J Orthod 55:585–599, 1969.
31. Stöckli PW, Teuscher UM: Combined activator headgear orthopedics. *In* Graber TM, Swain BF (eds.): Current Orthodontic Principles and Techniques. St. Louis, MO, C. V Mosby, 1985, pp. 405–483.
32. Tweed CH: Indications for extraction of teeth in orthodontic procedure. Am J Orthod Oral Surg 30:405–428, 1944.
33. Björk A, Skieller V: Postnatal growth and development of the maxillary complex. *In* McNamara JA Jr (ed.): Factors Affecting the growth of the Midface. Monograph no 6, Craniofacial Growth Series. Ann Arbor, MI, Center for Human Growth and Development, University of Michigan, 1976, pp. 61–99.
34. Thüer U, Ingervall B: Pressure from the lips on the teeth and malocclusion. Am J Orthod Dentofacial Orthop 90:234–242, 1986.
35. Solow B: The dentoalveolar compensatory mechanism: Background and clinical implications. Brit J Orthod 7:145–161, 1987.
36. Profitt WR: Equilibrium theory revisited. Angle Orthod 48:175–186, 1978.
37. Profitt WR: Lingual pressure patterns in the transition from tongue thrust to adult swallowing. Arch Oral Biol 17:555–563, 1975.
38. Nielsen IL: Maxillary superimposition: A comparison of three methods for cephalometric evaluation of growth and treatment change. Am J Orthod Dentofacial Orthop 95:422–431, 1989.

Considerations of Dentofacial Growth in Long-Term Retention and Stability

Ram S. Nanda
and
Surender K. Nanda

T he question of long-term retention and stability of occlusions after orthodontic treatment has always engaged the attention of the profession. The improvements achieved from long and painstaking treatment may be lost to varying degrees after the appliances are removed. Sometimes relapse in tooth positions is noted even during the period when an individual is using the retention appliances. A question often asked by patients and orthodontists is, How long should active retention with appliances be maintained?

Recent studies[1-3] on the assessment of long-term observations of posttreatment results have indicated that relapse occurred in most cases. Orthodontic treatment rendered in conjunction with extraction or nonextraction procedures met the same fate. No variable was found to be predictive of either stability or relapse.[4] Contemporary orthodontics has no satisfactory solution to the problem of achieving long-term stability.

A central question in the famous extraction/nonextraction debates of Case and Angle was the stability of the orthodontic treatment. Case challenged Angle's philosophy that nature always starts out to build a perfect denture in each individual and that malocclusions are caused by local factors. On the other hand, Case promoted the theory of biological variation and inheritance in the development of malocclusions. Case pleaded for extractions of first premolars in the treatment of patients with certain types of Angle Class II, Division 1 and bimaxillary protrusion malocclusions. Case stated in reply to his critics that "upon no basis but the bible theory of special creation can I reconcile the teaching that nature puts teeth into an individual's mouth that do not belong to his or her physiognomy."[5]

The debate on extraction versus nonextraction orthodontic treatment approaches has continued throughout this century. The matter of long-term stability of the corrected result has never been resolved. Several additional factors may have an important bearing on orthodontic stability. Among them are the influence of growth changes of dentofacial structures, balanced occlusion, and harmonious orofacial musculature. This chapter focuses on the effect of growth changes of the dentofacial structures on retention and stability of treated dentitions.

DENTOFACIAL SKELETAL CHANGES WITH GROWTH

Relapse of the corrected position of the teeth after successful orthodontic treatment is fully recognized by the clinician; however, skeletal changes that may occur during retention may attenuate, exaggerate, or maintain the dentoskeletal relationship. Relapse of the teeth is a source of annoyance, whereas an undesirable outcome of skeletal changes in the patient is left to the fate of the individual's so-called growth pattern. It is interesting to note that the clinical manifestations of skeletal relationships are given considerable importance at the initiation and during orthodontic treatment, but little or no consideration is given to posttreatment skeletal changes due to growth and their effect on the final outcome. This attitude is based on two assumptions. First, it is assumed that the responsibility for skeletal supervision is secondary to the dental relationships during active treatment. Further, when teeth are brought into proper interdigitation, the treatment is completed regardless of the skeletal maturation status of the individual. Second, it is assumed that not much can be done during the posttreatment phase to modify the growth pattern of the individual. The truth of the matter is that many patients at the completion of orthodontic treatment may still be going through the pubertal growth spurt and yet there may be others who have not even entered the period of accelerated pubertal growth.

Failure to recognize the continuing effect of dentofacial growth after the completion of orthodontic treatment and its resultant favorable or unfavorable effects on the physiognomy of the face and its dental relationships may jeopardize long-term stability of the orthodontic result.

The clinician often assumes at the completion of treatment that future skeletal growth is of no consequence or that dentofacial changes will be proportional and thus will maintain the skeletal relationships that were established during treatment. For many of our patients, orthodontic treatment is completed before skeletal growth has ceased; this observation is of particularly greater significance in boys than in girls since boys generally mature later. The major focus during retention is placed on the maintenance of the corrected positions of the teeth, and no compensations are made for the future dentoalveolar and skeletal growth of the jaws in either the horizontal or vertical direction.

What is suggested here is that retention devices should be differentially selected based upon the dentofacial morphology and the anticipated magnitude and directions of growth instead of the clinician simply using his or her favorite retention appliance.

The effect of continued growth after successful treatment is critical in individuals with short face syndrome.[6,7] These individuals may require dentoalveolar compensations (anterior bite plate) during the retention phase until maxillo-mandibular growth is completed. Failure to recognize the dominant horizontal pattern of growth of the individual may result in a "dished-in face" with or without extractions of teeth. Imagine the additional soft tissue growth, particularly in the noses of patients with deep bite and short vertical facial height. These individuals will have further exaggeration of their concave facial pattern. In contrast, individuals with long face syndrome may require a high-pull facebow headgear to hold the position of molars and to prevent further dentoalveolar growth and worsening of facial physiognomy. In some cases, even the dental relationships of the teeth resulted in noticeable relapse of dental open bite due to lack of ramal growth or excessive vertical dentoalveolar growth. It is obvious that post-treatment retention should be determined on the basis of dentofacial morphology rather than by the routine use of standard retention devices.

Of particular clinical significance is the timing of the pubertal growth spurt in individuals who manifest severe skeletal dysplasia (Fig. 2–1). The timing of the pubertal growth spurt between open bite and deep bite individuals within each sex is the same as is usually recognized between males and females. However, the pubertal growth spurt in skeletal deep-bite patients within each sex is shifted $1\frac{1}{2}$ to 2 years later than in patients with open bite. These individuals will require a longer retention period in contrast to the skeletal open bite subjects.

It is recognized that the mandible continues to grow until the late teen years, although this may not happen in all individuals. It is clinically observed that in severe Class II cases where the maxilla is protrusive (large anteroposteriorly), it continues to grow for a longer period, whereas the mandible may be experiencing little or no growth. This may alter the spatial relationships of the dental arches. In this situation it may be appropriate to maintain the anteroposterior position of the maxilla with a high-pull facebow headgear.[8] This retention device will prevent dentoalveolar growth of the maxillary molars and may in some instances improve facial configuration.

The point is that the clinician has to be alert to the growth pattern of an individual patient. Routine use of average values as a standard by which to measure deviations in size and maturational status of various dentofacial parameters for orthodontic diagnosis and treatment planning

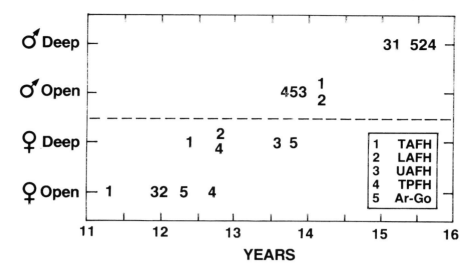

FIGURE 2–1   Schematic representation showing the timing of the peak of the pubertal spurts for five facial dimensions in open and deep bite subjects. (From Nanda SK: Patterns of vertical growth in the face. Am J Orthod 93:103–116, 1988.)

has lulled most clinicians into thinking that the patient will or is expected to follow an average pattern. The suitable treatment plans are developed using mean numbers assigned to a group of measurements. However, longitudinal growth studies have always emphasized the importance of variations among individuals as well as the various parameters within the same individual. Figure 2–2 shows a comparison of the dimensions of the sella-gnathion and nasion-gnathion in 10 individuals. Early- and late-maturing individuals are chronologically arranged and show tremendous variation. No single individual follows the peaks and valleys of the median curve. Peaks and valleys of individuals will tend to average out the fluctuations. The resulting average curve provides us with a central trend, but represents no single individual, and the impact of peaks and valleys has been diminished by the method of averaging.

It appears that the biologic variations in a population are large and difficult to fully fathom. A clinician may capitulate as deviant growth pattern what really are deviations from the so-called averages available from various atlases.[9–13] It is our belief that the longitudinal studies which have dealt with the data on a cross-sectional basis in developing the "normal" or average values have presented a far too simplistic approach to a very complex problem. Although prediction of facial growth pattern in its various dimensions belies our present knowledge, it is of critical importance to recognize this fact rather than to ignore it.

The duration and magnitude of the circumpubertal growth vary among individuals and even within the same individual. The age at which

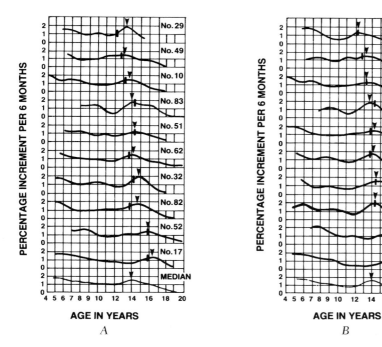

FIGURE 2–2   Comparison of dimensions of the sella-gnathion (A) and nasion-gnathion (B) in 10 individuals. Early- and late-maturing individuals are chronologically arranged and show tremendous variation in the timing of pubertal maximum. The arrow indicates the timing of the pubertal maximum peak growth for each individual measurement. Note also that the pubertal maximum for each measurement occurs at different times, and in the chronological order of sequence the position of an individual may vary. Nanda also reported similar observations on other facial dimensions. No single individual follows the peaks and valleys of the median incremental growth curve. Peaks and valleys of individuals tend to average out the fluctuations. The resulting median curve (bottom of each figure) provides us with a central trend, but represents no single individual, and the impact of peaks and valleys has been diminished by the method of averaging. (From Nanda RS: The rates of growth of several facial components measured from serial cephalometric roentgenograms. Am J Orthod 41:658–673, 1955.)

each individual, and, for that matter, each particular facial dimension, reaches the adult size depends on the individual's own pattern of physical growth and maturation. Take, for example, the longitudinal facial records of the two men shown in Figure 2–3. Five linear measurements of their faces have been highlighted in a group of 10 cases. Note that 32 had a relatively small facial length at the age of 4 years, its size remained rather small relative to the facial lengths of other members of the group even at age 19 years, and its rank was consistent with respect to the other nine individuals. On the other hand, 83 has a relatively large sella-gnathion

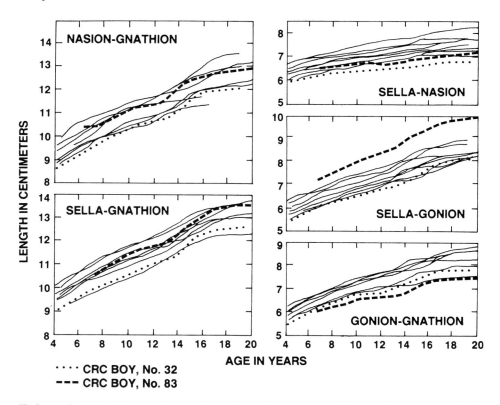

FIGURE 2–3 Comparisons of absolute dimensions of 2 men in a group of 10. (From Nanda RS: The rates of growth of several facial components measured from serial cephalometric roentgenograms. Am J Orthod 41:658–673, 1955.)

and nasion-gnathion, but a small sella-nasion and gonion-gnathion. His sella-gonion is the largest and his gonion-gnathion is the smallest in the group, thus giving this individual a long face that is proportionately small in depth. Note that his sella-gonion was still growing at age 20.

If we superimpose the relative increment curves on the same age scale for their different measurements, as in Figure 2–4, it is apparent that each dimension has a different rate of growth. In the case of 32, the gonion-gnathion grows at a relatively greater rate between the ages of 5 and 9 years, but during adolescence, the sella-gonion picks up the momentum and continues to exhibit more growth. In contrast, 83 showed greater circumpubertal growth in the gonion-gnathion than in all the other measurements, and the onset and maximum of pubertal spurt in this dimension was later than all the rest. However, between the ages of 17 and 18 years this individual experienced larger and continuing growth in the sella-gonion.

Many of these changes may continue even into the twenties for some individuals. Growth studies by Nanda[14–16] and Nanda et al[17] have shown that, particularly in males, growth in facial skeleton and soft tis-

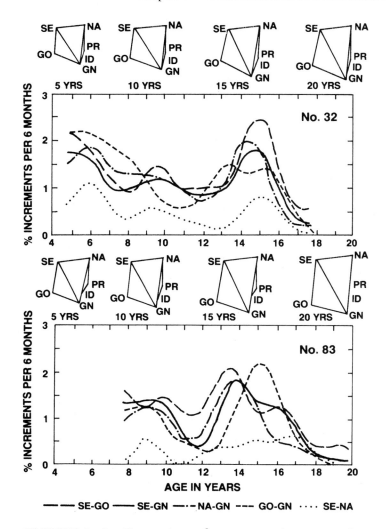

FIGURE 2–4   Comparison of percentage increments in two men, three-point smoothed twice. (From Nanda RS: The rates of growth of several facial components measured from serial cephalometric roentgenograms. Am J Orthod 41:658–673, 1955.)

sues continues past the age of 18 years. Even a change in size of 1 to 2 mm during the postpubertal years may have a profound effect on the long-term stability of an orthodontic treatment result.

SUMMARY

It is extremely important to pay attention to the individual's growth pattern, and a distinction must be made in the selection of retention devices based upon the nature and extent of dentofacial dysplasia (growth pattern). The duration of retention should depend upon the maturation status of the patient and anticipated future growth.

There is some merit in the philosophy of those clinicians who advocate permanent retention. Without being aware of the biomechanics of growth change, with their retention appliances, they are in fact carrying the patient through the active stages of growth.

Finally, one may philosophize that nothing about human morphology is stationary. Aging is a well-documented process of change. Dentitional adjustment and changing dental relationships are known to all even in otherwise healthy individuals. Then why do we expect long-term stability in every case? Perhaps the answer to the question of long-term stability is long-term retention.

REFERENCES

1. Little RM, Wallen TR, Riedel RA: Stability and relapse of mandibular anterior alignment—First premolar extraction cases treated by traditional edgewise orthodontics. Am J Orthod 80:349–365, 1981.
2. Little RM, Riedel RA, Artun J: An evaluation of changes in mandibular anterior alignment from 10 to 20 years postretention. Am J Orthod 93:423–428, 1988.
3. Little RM, Riedel RA: Postretention evaluation of stability and relapse—Mandibular arches with generalized spacing. Am J Orthod 95:37–41, 1989.
4. Shields TE, Little RM, Chapko MK: Stability and relapse of mandibular anterior alignment: A cephalometric appraisal of first-premolar extraction cases treated by traditional edgewise orthodontics. Am J Orthod 87:27–38, 1985.
5. Case CS: The question of extraction in orthodontia. Dent Cosmos 54:137–57, 276–284, 1912.
6. Nanda SK: Patterns of vertical growth in the face. Am J Orthod 93:103–116, 1988.
7. Nanda SK: Circumpubertal growth spurt related to vertical dysplasia. Angle Orthod 59:113–122, 1990.
8. Nanda SK: Growth patterns in subjects with long and short faces. Am J Orthod, in press.
9. Riedel RA: The relation of maxillary structures to cranium in malocclusion and in normal occlusion. Angle Orthod 22:142–145, 1952.
10. Downs WB: Variations in facial relationships: Their significance in treatment and prognosis. Am J Orthod 34:812–840, 1948.
11. Steiner CC: Cephalometrics for you and me. Am J Orthod 39:729–755, 1953.
12. Steiner CC: Cephalometrics in clinical practice. Angle Orthod 29:8–29, 1959.
13. Riolo ML, Moyers RE, McNamara JA, Hunter WS: An Atlas of Craniofacial Growth: Cephalometric Standards from the University School Growth Study. Monograph No. 2, Craniofacial Growth Series. Ann Arbor, MI, Center for Human Growth and Development, University of Michigan, 1974.

14. Nanda RS: The rates of growth of several facial components measured from serial cephalometric roentgenograms. Am J Orthod 41:658–673, 1955.
15. Nanda RS: Cephalometric study of the human face from serial roentgenograms. Ergebnisse Der Anatomie und Entwicklungs-Geschichte 35:358–419, 1956.
16. Nanda RS: Growth changes in skeletal-facial profile and their significance in orthodontic diagnosis. Am J Orthod 59:501–513, 1971.
17. Nanda RS, Meng H, Kapila S, Goorhuis J: Growth changes in the soft tissue profile. Angle Orthod 60:177–190, 1990.

Perspectives in Orthodontic Stability

Charles J. Burstone

Among the goals of orthodontic treatment beyond facial and dental aesthetics, function, and the health and longevity of the dentition is the achievement of stable or relatively stable results. Anecdotally, one can hear at orthodontic meetings extreme positions on the stability of orthodontic patients. Some clinicians will say that a well-treated case by certain criteria or a specific technique will always lead to stability and, therefore, that stability is really no problem. At the other extreme, others will claim that no matter what you do, extract or not extract, expand or not expand, most treatment is bound to lead to failure. To support this uncomfortable latter position, there have recently appeared in the literature studies of the outcomes of orthodontic treatment that suggest a higher degree of relapse than optimistically might be anticipated.[1-3]

The reality of our present knowledge is that no form of treatment guarantees absolute stability, nor does a well-treated case treated by the highest standards by itself assure stability. This does not suggest, since we do not know all of the many factors that produce instability, that our treatment goals must ignore a stable occlusion and that permanent retention is inevitable. This chapter examines the factors that may influence the long-term stability of patients so that our treatment goals and mechanics may be improved.

What is a stable dentition? The answer to this question is not so obvious. Teeth after orthodontic treatment are not ankylosed to the bone. The periodontal ligament is part of the adjustment mechanisms of the stomatognathic system, which allows teeth to migrate under changing conditions. The work of Björk with metallic implants has well documented that teeth migrate as the skeletal pattern changes with growth.[4,5,6] Even in nongrowing adults migrations occur. There exists a relationship between functional occlusion and the pattern of tooth migration, and as teeth wear, or periodontal support is lost, there may be further migration of teeth. If one compares on study models the occlusion following treatment with the occlusion after the retention period, the occlusions might superficially look identical. Most likely, however, considerable migration of teeth has occurred within the respective jaw bones. So stability does not mean that the teeth have not moved but rather that we have maintained certain goals of static and functional occlusion.

We should more properly compare the stability of finished cases with the stability of untreated normals. There is much variation in what happens with untreated patients, but certain secular trends might be mentioned. Much has been written about the crowding of the lower incisors, which is a natural occurrence that can be found in untreated patients.[7] Only if we have more crowding than expected after retention can it be assumed that the treatment result is unstable. Although the reasons for crowding of lower anterior teeth may be debated, the orthodontist should consider this possibility in guiding his treatment goals. If the diagnosis of a given patient suggests that more crowding will occur even after a good end result, this should be compensated for by modifying treatment goals and procedures.

Inevitably we come to the conclusion that stability is not an absolute, and what one tries to do for a patient is to obtain acceptable stability. The concept of acceptable stability is not an alibi for treatment but a recognition of biological limitations. The success of our treatment should be measured based upon some type of ratio between the magnitude of patient improvement and the relapse. If the ratio is not very high, one could question how wise orthodontic treatment was for the patient.

$$\text{Success Index} = \frac{\text{Magnitude of Improvement}}{\text{Magnitude of Relapse}}$$

The typical type of orthodontic relapse is well documented.[8–10] It includes crowding or spacing of teeth, return of deep overbite or open bite, instability of the Class II and Class III correction, instability of subdivision cases, and general return of malalignment. One troubling aspect of relapse has been the overemphasis on lower incisor crowding, since part of the problem might be related to inherent growth changes and functional changes that might occur anyway. This chapter emphasizes factors that look more broadly at relapse rather than the special problem of the lower anterior teeth.

The broader view suggests that we look at many factors that can influence the stability of the dentition. There has been a tendency to develop popular and simplistic theories that offer convenient goals for treatment. Hence, we might read or hear that if we place the teeth in excellent occlusion the case will be stable, or that if we position the lower incisor to some cephalometric standard, stability is ensured. Obviously, instability has multiple causes, and the orthodontist should avoid simplistic explanations. Rather than discuss all of the anatomical and functional factors that conceivably could lead to stability, this chapter selects just a few and discusses their relationship in reaching the orthodontist's goal of greater stability of the finished result.

NORMAL GROWTH, ORTHOPEDIC CHANGES, AND RELAPSE

Typically, the mandible grows and displaces forward at a faster rate than the maxilla (measured to occlusal plane). Tooth compensations include the tendency of the lower incisors to move lingually. If after treatment the lower incisor is in a precarious position (perhaps it has been flared), more than average mandibular growth during and after treatment could be a contributing factor to crowding in the lower anterior region.

Treatment is simplified and success more easily assured in Class II patients who exhibit significant mandibular growth. If growth is more limited, treatment might have the effect of retracting the upper posterior teeth. Often molars are tipped distally and are not in the most stable position because they tend to come forward with time. This treatment result could become stable if during the retention and postretention period favorable mandibular growth occurs. If there is sufficient forward growth of the mandible, upper molars can come forward and assume better axial inclinations and more room would be available posteriorly for the eruption of second and third molars.

Unfortunately, the typical growth that helps treatment in the Class II patient works against the correction of a Class III case. It is not very uncommon to have a Class III occlusion corrected by eruption of posterior teeth (Class III elastics or protraction headgear) and for the mandible to rotate back to its original position in time. The patient may be told that the Class III is recurring because of an abnormal amount of mandibular growth. This may not be the case, as shown in Figure 3–1, where the mandible was rotated downward and backward during treatment but relapsed later on. Figure 3–1A shows the changes during the initial phase of treatment, which lasted 10 months. Although the patient exhibited a convex face, the A-B to occlusion plane relationship demonstrated a Class III denture base relationship. Before treatment molars were Class III; the incisors that were spaced had normal overjet; and posteriors were in crossbite.

Treatment included closure of the incisor spacing, maxillary expansion to correct the crossbite, and Class III elastics to correct the Class III occlusion. Treatment results appeared dramatic. The Class III occlusion was corrected, and overbite and overjet increased. The separate maxillary

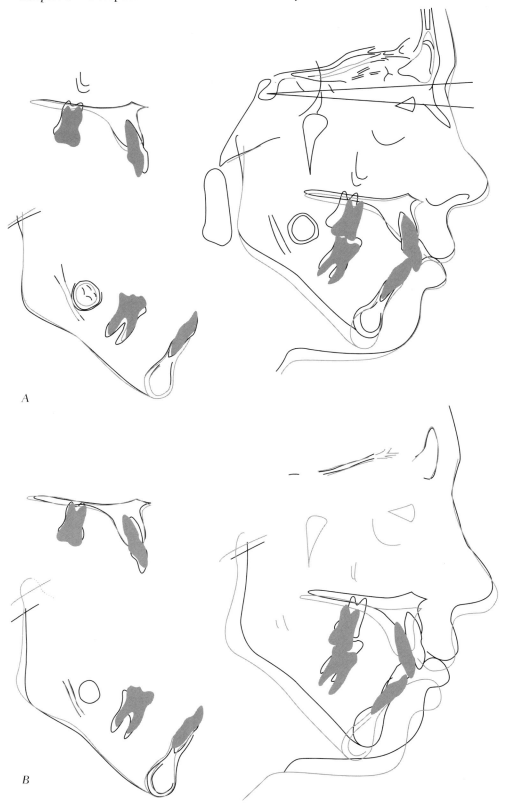

A

B

FIGURE 3–1   *(See opposite page for legend.)*

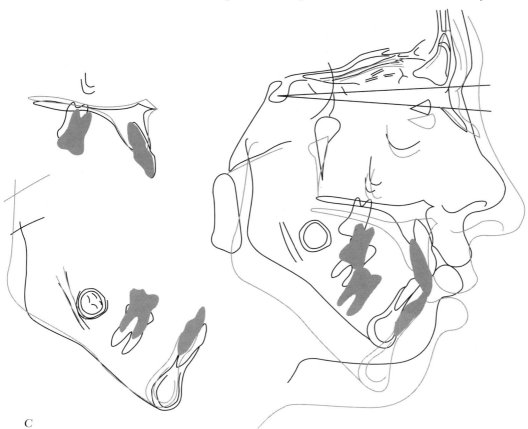

C

FIGURE 3–1   Class III patient nonsurgical and nonextraction treatment. *A,* Changes after first phase of treatment: Class III corrected by hinging open the mandible. *B,* Second phase of treatment: continued downward and backward rotation of the mandible. *C,* 3 years, 3 months after treatment. The patient has relapsed into Class III. The mandible has rotated in a counterclockwise direction. The mandibular growth is small and not responsible for the relapse.

and mandibular superimpositions show that the upper incisors were retracted and the lower incisors remained in their original anteroposterro position. The retraction of the upper incisors should have led to underjet, but this did not happen because the extrusive mechanics on the posterior teeth rotated the mandible open. This rotation was also responsible for the correction of the Class III occlusion. Figure 3–1*B* shows the changes during a second phase of treatment, primarily directed at correcting the relapsed cross bite. During this 11-month phase, mandibular growth was present; however, the increments (Ar-Pg) were slightly less than average. The Class III correction remained stable because the mandible was rotated open even more by extrusion of the posteriors. Overjet was helped by some flaring of the upper incisors.

Figure 3–1*C* shows the changes 3 years 3 months after treatment. The patient returned with a pronounced 8-mm Class III molar occlusion and return of the cross bite. It was suggested to the patient that the relapse was not the fault of the orthodontist but was caused by "a large amount of mandibular growth that produced forward positioning of the lower jaw." This explanation does not correlate with the cephalometric findings. What happened was that the mandible was hinged open during treatment, giving a *pseudocorrection* of the Class III occlusion. The A-B to occlusal plane discrepancy was ignored in designing the treatment plan. Furthermore, if the increments (Ar-Pg) of mandibular growth are compared to standards, growth is less than average at every age. Following treatment, the mandible hinged back and the full Class III dental and skeletal problem that was always present expressed itself. Too often relapse of Class III cases is blamed on abnormal mandibular growth when the problem is that iatrogenic treatment rotates a mandible open. A stable correction of the patient shown in Figure 3–1 is better obtained by not rotating the mandible but by anteropostero *tooth movement* or surgical *bone* correction of the anteropostero discrepancy. Some patients with small vertical dimension and large interocclusal space can successfully be hinged open.

It should be recognized that growth is important not only during treatment but after treatment. It can either help or hinder us in achieving a stable result. Just looking at teeth on a study cast, either the original or the final, does not give the proper prospective of the dynamic migration changes that are occurring. As orthodontists, we should stop using the alibi that our failure was due to a poor growth pattern. Our failure may be related to our inability to diagnose the problem properly or to anticipate normal growth changes, but rarely to some unusual growth pattern. The two most common alibis for orthodontic failure are poor growth pattern and lack of patient cooperation. If we are able to consider the growth potential of our patient during treatment and after, we will have better insight into how to achieve long-term stability.

A great deal of argument still centers on how much of an orthopedic change is produced in orthodontic treatment. For example, in treating Class II cases it appears that most of the changes which occur are related to normal growth, but superimposed on the normal growth may be some small orthopedic changes. Long-term outcome studies that are beginning to be reported suggest that orthopedic changes may be found during the first few years of treatment, but over the long term there may be no significant difference between untreated Class II patients and those undergoing so-called orthopedic treatment with functional appliances or fixed appliances like the Herbst.[10,11] One might suggest that this rebound toward the original skeletal configuration adds to the overall instability of the case; thus, a Class II case can relapse because the teeth move or because the maxilla may come forward a little more than normal if it has been orthopedically retruded; the mandible may also demonstrate less growth in the posttreatment period if it temporarily grew more because of an orthopedic effect during treatment.

STABILITY AND MANDIBULAR ROTATION DURING TREATMENT

Studies have shown that there is a high incidence of relapse in patients with deep overbite. A number of factors may be at work to explain relapse in the deep overbite case. In growers as well as nongrowers, extrusive mechanics involving the posterior teeth can produce rotation and hinging open of the mandible, with two possible mechanisms for the relapse. First, the mandible could rotate closed with a concomitant increase in deep overbite. Second, the increased vertical dimension may maintain itself. With the increase in vertical dimension, a large interlabial gap may be produced with larger lip pressures (if the patient has a closed habitual lip posture). Furthermore, there may be an increase in cheek pressure in the cuspid region associated with the increase in vertical dimension. These lip pressures can lead to crowding of the lower anteriors with an increase in overjet, which causes the deep overbite to return.

It is important in patients with powerful masticatory musculature associated with small anterior vertical dimension to correct the deep overbite by intrusion of anterior teeth. If extrusive mechanics on posterior teeth are used, the appliances should be left in place until the anteriors and posteriors have been intruded and the original vertical dimension established. Posterior extrusion is possible and stable if sufficient growth is present.

In growing patients, as the mandible descends vertically more than the maxilla, there can be room for the eruption of posterior teeth. However, if too much eruption occurs from improper mechanics, the mandible will hinge open. During the retention period it is important to maintain the position of the teeth while the mandible continues to grow. In postretention tracings the mandible typically will be seen to rotate in a counterclockwise manner, with the gonion moving further inferior than the pogonion and with a flattening of the occlusal plane. Retention in both arches (removable or fixed) is necessary to prevent crowding until growth has corrected the hinging open of the mandible. After growth has caught up with the supereruption of the posterior teeth, overbite correction should be more stable.

If a Class II, Division I or Division II patient exhibits deep overbite, extrusion of the posterior teeth while the mandible grows usually leads to a reasonably stable correction. On the other hand, if there is not sufficient growth, mechanics leading to the intrusion of anteriors must be employed. There is now a growing strong body of evidence to suggest that intrusion of incisors offers a more stable method of correction of deep overbite than overly extruding posterior teeth.[12,13]

Related to the relapse of deep overbite cases is the opposite condition—the open bite. Patients with a divergent skeletal pattern (a palatomandibular angle greater than average) commonly exhibit upper and lower occlusal planes that are not parallel but diverge anteriorly. Improper orthodontic treatment can exaggerate these two occlusal planes. Examples include leveling an upper arch with central incisors superior to the posterior teeth, which can flatten the upper plane and increase the divergence. Even more deleterious is any extrusion of posterior teeth that causes the mandible to hinge open and produce divergence of the two occlusal planes. The increase in vertical dimension associated with posterior extrusion, the anterior open bite that is produced, and the ensuing tongue seal add to the problem of open bite correction and its stability. Maxillary impaction carried out surgically by Lefort I procedures has been shown to be particularly stable as a solution to skeletal open bites; nevertheless, not all skeletal problems will be treated by surgery. Some are borderline, and, therefore, careful mechanics must be used not to alter the parallelism of the occlusal planes unfavorably and not to increase the vertical dimension.

ARCH WIDTH AND STABILITY

Historically, there has been great interest in the possibility of expanding cuspid width for solving arch length inadequacies. Since the cuspid is around the corner of the arch, any increase in cuspid width can dramatically lead to increases in arch length.

Cuspid width has most commonly been increased by dental expansion. Some clinicians claim that the use of functional shields or lip bumpers produce expansion by altering the underlining apical base. Definitive evidence at this time has not been forthcoming to suggest that the basal bone is actually expanded with these appliances. The axial inclination of teeth may appear less tipped with the use of shields and bumpers because they allow teeth to erupt in many instances along their long axis. By contrast, dental expansion, usually with single forces, will move crowns in one direction buccally and the roots toward the lingual. Another approach to cuspid expansion is the use of rapid palatal expansion in the maxillary arch, which has been demonstrated to produce permanent width changes in the maxilla with the hope that lower cuspid widths would be stable in a wider configuration.[14] Most studies have shown that changes in lower cuspid width subsequent to maxillary expansion are relatively small. Since our ability to expand skeletally the mandibular apical base is limited, our attention should now be drawn to the possibilities of altering intercuspid width dentally and to evaluate some of our limitations in doing so.

What determines the stability of cuspid width? It has been thought that there is a balance of forces between the cheek and the tongue. This equilibrium concept is a gross oversimplification, since experimental work shows that tongue pressures, particularly during swallowing, are much greater than cheek pressures.[15] The equilibrium that is present is related more to an energy concept where time is a factor. Many forces operate on the cuspids, not only the intermittent tongue forces or the more constant cheek forces but also the forces of occlusion. A working hypothesis might be that if the cuspid is moved too far into the cheek, the constant cheek pressures will tend to return the cuspid from whence it came.

A guiding principle commonly used in orthodontics is that the original cuspid width is inviolate. Should we use the original width as a reasonable guide for a final stable arch? It is true that in untreated cases after the full eruption of the cuspid, the average cuspid width does not increase but may actually narrow. One of the difficulties in treating to the original cuspid width is that the concept is a static one which does not consider many important factors that will now be discussed.

The effect of growth, both skeletal and neuromuscular, on arch width and arch form is not thoroughly understood; however, depending upon the amount of differential growth (including rotation between the maxilla and mandible), compensations occur in the direction of tooth eruption that can alter arch form. For instance, in backward rotators the lower incisors and the cuspids can move distally in respect to the mandible. Does this mean that cuspids can assume a wider width in these patients? The answer is not obvious, since at the same time neuromuscular adaptations are occurring. There is a greater anterior vertical dimension in the backward-rotating patients in comparison to the forward rotators. This could lead to tighter cheek musculature and limit an increase in cuspid width. The reverse is true with the forward rotator. In short, we do not know much about relating growth to arch widths.

In theory, a patient undergoing extraction therapy should be able to accommodate a wider cuspid width, since the cuspids are moving posteriorly in a wider part of the arch. Then why do cuspids narrow even in extraction cases in which the original cuspid widths have been preserved? The original cuspid widths may be misleading because in some arch length inadequacies cuspids are blocked out labially. Such a blocked-out cuspid should not be used to establish the correct width for the patient; it is little wonder that when arches are expanded to this original width relapse can occur. Sometimes it is not recognized that the intercuspid width dimension may not reflect the arch form required for the patient. A cuspid, for example, may be blocked out on one side alone. The proper narrowing of cuspid width should be performed on one side only. If the original cuspid widths were used in this situation, the cuspid position on the stable side might be jeopardized.

A number of neuromuscular factors should be considered in establishing cuspid widths. Many of them, unfortunately, are not fully understood. If a patient has a wide interoral slit, so that the oral aperture is found distal to the cuspid, the break in the wraparound muscle sheet at the corner of the mouth can give greater freedom in modifying or expanding cuspid widths.

A clinical evaluation of the tightness of the cheek and its position relative to the cuspid in rest position can also be useful. Typically, in rest position the occlusal one third of the mandibular cuspid is not covered by the soft tissues of the cheek. Some patients exhibit deep overbite in the cuspid region where the lower cuspids have been locked lingually and where they are positioned far away from the cheek musculature. In these patients it may be possible to expand the lower cuspids to fit the maxillary arch. In other patients, when the lower cuspid is covered over by the cheek, expansion may not be feasible because of the tight musculature.

If during treatment the vertical dimension is increased by hinging the mandible open, the greater cheek tension could be responsible for narrowing the dental arches. This creates a retention problem, since these pressures can lead to crowding in the arches. With further muscular and skeletal growth, the mandibular rotational changes may disappear, and a wider or more normal cuspid width may be stable.

In summary, when we try to establish what the cuspid width should be at the end of treatment and what our limitations are in dental expansion, the orthodontist must consider all of his knowledge and experience in diagnosis and treatment planning; simple guidelines are not sufficient. Such statements as, "One can expand with a shield or lip bumper" or "One cannot change widths and must maintain the original intercuspid width" are dangerous simplifications.

INCISOR POSITION AND STABILITY

Some orthodontic relapse is related to a change in the anteropostero position of the incisors. In order to establish a stable position for the incisors, a number of dogmas have developed. These dogmas may have merit in that they force the clinician to identify specific treatment goals. Let us now examine three commonly stated dogmas.

It has been stated and widely accepted that the most stable position for a lower incisor is a cephalometric mean. Means have been established in a number of studies of subjects with either desirable faces or good occlusions. From the point of view of facial aesthetics there is large variation in the positioning of the incisor, and the same is true in selecting samples with excellent occlusion. For example, the lower incisor to mandibular plane, which averages about 90°, may have a standard deviation of 5°. Within 2 standard deviations in 95 percent of a population of normals a variation of ±10°, or ±20° total variation is found. This would also be true for the lower incisor inclination to Frankfort horizontal, which may have a standard deviation of 4.5° and hence a variation at the 95 percent confidence level of 18°. Picking a measurement that relates the lower incisor to the maxilla and mandible (lower incisor to A-Pogonion), the 2° standard deviation gives a plus or minus variation of 4 mm, or a total variation of 8 mm. When a normal sample varies as much as 8 mm in the positioning of a lower incisor, the mean does not give much of a guide for positioning the incisor. The same result is found for any cephalometric standard. It must be noted that in all of the above samples the subjects have stable occlusions, and there is no evidence that being closer to the mean is any more stable than being farther away. Considering the lower incisor to A-Pogonion within 3 standard deviations, one would find a total of 12 mm of variation in the position of the incisor. Furthermore, the orthodontist treats patients who do not have normal occlusions but who have skeletal variation. It has been well documented that in patients with skeletal variation and normal occlusion there is an even greater variation in the position of the incisors. For example, in a prognathic patient lower incisors tend to compensate by leaning lingually. And in many Class II skeletal patterns, because of the lack of restraint of the lip, the lower incisor can lean to the labial.

A second dogma states that the best position for the lower incisor is its original position. It is true that the original malocclusion could be a stable position for the lower incisor. The correction of the malocclusion, however, may place that relatively stable incisor in a nonstable position. For example, the lower lip caught between the upper and lower incisors flares the upper incisor and may retrude the lower incisor in a Class II, Division I patient. At the end of treatment lower lip pressures may allow some protrusion of the lower anteriors from their original positions. In many Class III patients a tight lower lip produces forces retracting and crowding the lower incisors. The more stable position of the lower anteriors could be farther back than the pretreatment position if no surgery is planned.

A third dogma states that there is only one stable position of the lower incisor. Clinical experience suggests that there are many stable positions. In fact, the original malocclusion may be the most stable position of them all. The lip and the tongue may adapt to the tooth position, and the teeth may adapt to the pressures of the musculature. We are left with the inescapable conclusion that there may be multiple positions of stability and that, unfortunately, in some patients no stable position can be found that meets the goals of a corrected malocclusion.

As with the determination of arch widths, simplistic explanations cannot take the place of good diagnosis and treatment planning. Even though we do not know all of the answers concerning the stability of the A-P position of the anterior teeth, it is necessary to make judgments based on skeletal, neuromuscular, and functional factors.

INTRA-ARCH FACTORS AND STABILITY

Some of the relapse in Class II malocclusions in which spacing or flaring occurs, rotations return, and the intermaxillary correction relapses may be attributed to transseptal and gingival fibers. These problems can be minimized by early correction of rotations and other types of tooth-to-tooth alignment, overtreatment of tooth-to-tooth problems by overrotation, and in cases of space disclosure, root movement into an extraction site. Fiberotomies may be helpful, but they should not replace good treatment procedures, which include early treatment and overcorrection.[16] Recognition that it may take some time for soft tissues to adjust suggests that some retention may be required for lengthy periods of time until soft tissue remodeling has been completed. The rationale for soft tissue remodeling retention has a better biological base than holding teeth with retainers in muscularly unstable positions.

Intra-arch considerations go beyond awareness of transseptal and gingival fibers. Good contact areas and the reshaping of contact areas so that forces can be better distributed throughout the arch may be important considerations, particularly when lip pressures exert strong forces lingually on lower incisors.

FUNCTIONAL OCCLUSION AND STABILITY

One of the continuing discussions in dentistry is what is the proper relationship of the jaws in full occlusion—that is, centric relation. Some may define the ideal position as the mandible in its most retruded or boundary position. Although physiologically the boundary position may not be the ideal, it could serve as a guide for most of our orthodontic treatment. A long centric of 0.5 to 1 mm from the retruded position certainly is acceptable. Some treated Class II cases may end up with two intercuspal positions (Sunday bite). This loss of a definitive centric should be considered relapse. The use of Class II and Class III elastics for asymmetries may temporarily shift the jaw so it appears that a unilateral Class II is corrected. Later on the mandible returns to its original position, and the asymmetry fully or in part reasserts itself. The success of an orthodontic patient cannot be evaluated only in centric occlusion; but centric relation using a broad definition must be achieved.

Recent attention has been concentrated on the relationship between functional occlusion and symptoms related to the temporomandibular joint. Equally important is functional occlusion and its role in the stability of the dentition. An interesting study was carried out by Beyron in Sweden on a group of adult subjects who were followed longitudinally for many years.[17] His conclusions were very intriguing and suggest directions of future research. He found that patients who exhibited multidirectional chewing (patients who chewed on both right and left sides and protruded during incision) had minimal migration of teeth. On the other hand, in patients with deep overbites who were mainly bilateral chewers there was migration in the bicuspid and cuspid region. The patients that were sagittal chewers, easily protruding their jaws but locking them laterally, tended to show some flaring of the upper incisors. Figure 3–2 from Beyron shows a dentition with predominantly sagittal movements. The eight-year period

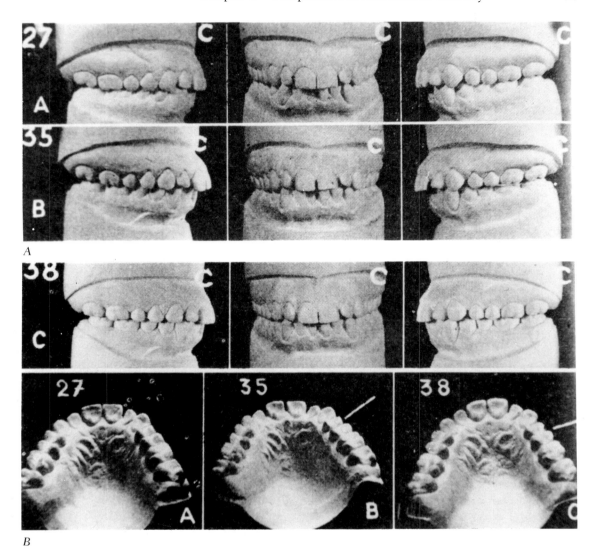

FIGURE 3–2 Adult patient: no history of orthodontics. The individual is functionally a sagittal chewer without lateral movements. From *A* to *B*, ages 27–35, the upper incisors tipped labially. Note the diastema between the incisors. After the bicuspids were equilibrated at age 35 to allow lateral movement, the diastema spontaneously closed. *C*, Age 38 years. (From Beyron HL: Occlusal changes in adult dentition. JADA 48:674–686, 1954.)

from age 27 years to 35 years shows labial tipping of the maxillary incisors as well as some attrition.[17] After occlusal adjustment the diastema between the central incisors spontaneously closed. The patient was an adult without any history of orthodontic treatment. Figure 3–3, by contrast, shows another of Beyron's patients with no history of orthodontic treatment who had a relatively stable dentition from age 32 years to age

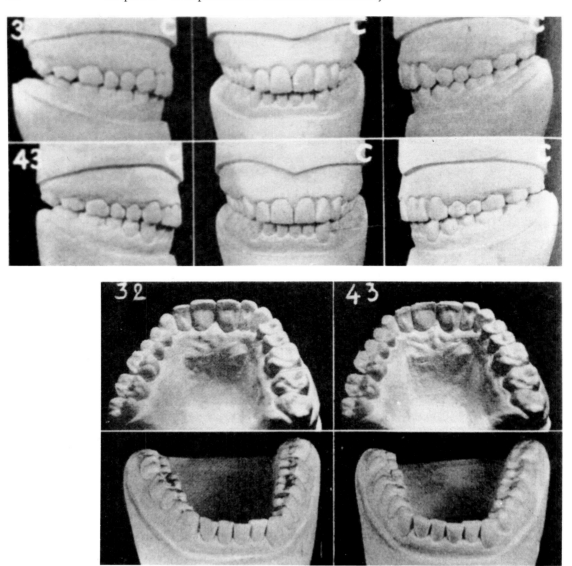

FIGURE 3–3   A dentition with multidirectional functional movements. Little migration of teeth is seen from ages 32 years to 43 years. Data from the study support the theory that multidirectional-functioning patients may be more stable. (From Beyron HL: Occlusal changes in adult dentition. JADA 48:674–686, 1954.)

43 years. This patient was characterized by multidirectional gliding movements. Other than some reduction in incisal guidance through wear, the dentition was relatively stable.

Beyron's classic study was published in 1954 and has not been given the attention it deserves. Although this study was small (44 patients) and was partly anecdotal, it is highly suggestive of future research that should focus on relating functional movements to dentition stability. If the study is confirmed, it implies that too much cuspid rise might lead to flaring of the upper incisors and crowding of the lower anteriors.

SUMMARY

There is no question that stability should be one of our major objectives in successfully treating an orthodontic patient. To reach this goal the orthodontist must have a realistic awareness of stability. Medicine has a better history of dealing with failure than dentistry does. Physicians know that patients die no matter what treatment procedures are used. In medicine, autopsies are routinely done to identify the cause of death. In dentistry, the tendency has been to hide failures in the closet. When failures are ignored or not documented, new generations of orthodontists are continually trained who believe that stability is no problem.

Ultimately, stability is related to the forces that act on the teeth, and hence it is a neuromuscular problem. In this sense morphology is secondary. However, with morphological changes teeth, bones, and muscles respond in different patterns and produce changes in the forces that act upon the teeth.

What causes the instability of orthodontic patients? Some factors have been discussed in this chapter, but there are countless others. Hence, stability is multivariate, and attempts to reduce it to simple goals, rules, and treatment techniques that guarantee stability are misguided.

The orthodontist may sometimes worry about stability at the time the retaining appliances are placed. Stability, however, really begins with the first clinical examination and includes a good data base and treatment plan. Specific treatment goals should be designed with stability in mind except in those few cases where no stable result is possible or where facial aesthetics might be compromised. Specific treatment goals must be followed with the appropriate treatment mechanics to reach the desired end so that proper positioning of bones and teeth in three-dimensional space, with consideration given to neuromuscular mechanisms, is achieved. Retention is part of stability, but there is more to retention than throwing in a lower cuspid-to-cuspid or an upper Hawley retainer. Retention is designed to maintain the occlusion during transitional phases of growth, during remodeling of soft tissue gingival and transseptal fibers, and during muscular adaptation. Retention is a continuation of treatment planning, and it requires the same kind of analytical thinking that is used to establish specific treatment objectives at the beginning of the case.

No, not all cases are stable, but neither are all cases unstable. Our lack of knowledge about all of the factors leading to stability should not deter us from keeping stability as one of our major objectives. It is certainly a worthy goal of this symposium to bring together some of the best minds in orthodontics to discuss stability, with its multivariate etiology, and to offer possible solutions for improving the stability and quality of treatment.

REFERENCES

1. Riedel RA: A review of the retention problem. Angle Orthod 30:179, 1960.
2. Riedel RA: Post-pubertal occlusal changes. *In* McNamara JA Jr (ed.): Factors Affecting the Growth Series. Ann Arbor, MI, Center for Human Growth and Development, University of Michigan, 1977, pp. 113–140.
3. Joondeph DR, Riedel RA: Retention. *In* Graber TM, Swain BF (eds.): Orthodontics: Principles and Techniques. St. Louis, MO, C. V. Mosby, 1985, pp. 857–898.
4. Björk A: Variations in the growth pattern of the human mandible: Longitudinal radiographic study by the implant method. J Dent Res 42:400–411, 1963.
5. Björk A: Sutural growth of the upper face studied by the implant method. Eur Orthod Soc Trans, pp. 49–65, 1964.
6. Lundstrom A: Changes in crowding and spacing of the teeth with age. Dent Pract 19:218, 1968.
7. Richardson ME: The role of the third molar in the case of late lower arch crowding: A review. Am J Orthod 95:79–83, 1989.
8. Shapiro PA, Kokich VG: The rationale of various models of retention. Symp Orthod Dent Clinics North America, 1981, pp 177–193.
9. Little RM, Wallen TR, Riedel RA: Stability and relapse of mandibular anterior alignment: First premolar extraction cases treated by traditional edgewise orthodontics. Am J Orthod 80:349, 1981.
10. Pancherz H: The nature of Class II relapse after Herbst appliance treatment: A cephalometric long-term investigation. Am J Orthod Dentofacial Orthop 100:220–233, 1991.
11. Devincenzo P: Changes in mandibular length before, during, and after successful orthopedic correction of Class II malocclusions using a functional appliance. Am J Orthod Dentofacial Orthop 99:241–255, 1991.
12. Burstone CJ: Deep overbite correction by intrusion. Am J Orthod 72(1):1–22, 1977.
13. Burzin J: The stability of deep overbite correction. Masters' thesis, Dept. of Orthodontics, University of Connecticut, 1991.
14. Isaacson RJ, Ingram AH: Forces produced by rapid maxillary expansion. II: Forces present during treatment. Angle Orthod 34:261, 1964.
15. Proffit WR: Equilibrium theory revisted, factors influencing position of the teeth. Angle Orthod, 48:175–186, 1978.
16. Edwards JG: A study of the periodontium during orthodontic rotation of teeth. Am J Orthod 30:14, 1960.
17. Beyron, HL: Occlusal changes in adult dentition. JADA 48:674–686, 1954.

The Stability of Deep Overbite Correction

Jeffrey Burzin
and
Ravindra Nanda

Correcting a deep bite can be accomplished by true intrusion of anterior teeth, extrusion of posterior teeth, or a combination of intrusion and extrusion. The type of tooth movement one chooses to employ is dependent upon the treatment objectives for the individual patient. Extrusion of posterior teeth may be the treatment of choice in growing patients if one wishes to increase lower face height, steepen the mandibular plane, correct lip redundancy, or increase facial convexity. However, this treatment is not appropriate for all patients; in fact, the stability of extrusion of posterior teeth has been questioned.

In many nonsurgical patients, intrusion of anterior teeth is the treatment of choice for correction of a deep bite. In patients exhibiting an excessive amount of maxillary incisors and gingiva, a large interlabial gap, a long lower facial height, or a steep mandibular plane, intrusion may be indicated. The method used to treat deep overbite should be determined by proper treatment planning, with consideration given to aesthetics, occlusal plane, lip competence, vertical skeletal dimension, skeletal convexity (the A-B discrepancy), and stability of the final result.

Numerous methods have been used to correct deep overbite. Hemley,[1] in 1938, described the use of the bite plate to retard the growth of the anterior alveolus and to allow the posterior alveolus to increase, thereby allowing for the eruption of the posterior teeth. He also found that only 1 patient out of 22 showed intrusion of the lower incisors. Strang[2] also stated that the bite plate elevates molars but has no anterior intrusive effect. Sleichter[3] studied the vertical changes of molars and incisors with bite-plane treatment. He found that alveolar height in the molar region increased while there was minimal change in the incisor area.

In edgewise therapy it is common to correct deep overbite by leveling the curve of Spee. This can be accomplished by an intrusion arch or by placing a continuous wire with a reverse curve of Spee (or an accentuated curve for the upper arch). The force system created by a reverse curve of Spee wires is such that an intrusive force is delivered to the incisors and an extrusive force is applied to the molars and premolars. Since extrusion is more easily accomplished than intrusion, a reverse curve of Spee wires will extrude posterior teeth while obtaining minimal, if any, anterior intrusion.[4] A study by Dake and Sinclair[5] showed that Tweed-type leveling arches using a reverse curve of Spee, tip-back bends, and step bends resulted in 0.3 mm of mean incisor extrusion

Another commonly used appliance to intrude incisors is the utility arch.[6] Studies of the utility arch show a range of 1 to 3 mm of true incisor intrusion.[5,7,8] Both the Dake[5] and Greig[7] studies showed that an average of about 1.1 mm of intrusion is possible with the utility arch, while Otto[8] showed an average of 2.0 mm of lower incisor intrusion and 0.55 mm of maxillary incisor intrusion.

BIOMECHANICS OF INTRUSION

Genuine intrusion of incisors can be accomplished with an intrusion base arch, as described by Burstone.[9] A study by Gottlieb[10] using the intrusion arch with forces ranging from 15 to 20 g per incisor showed that no measurable root shortening or visible blunting of the apexes occurred. Gottlieb showed that the mean intrusion in his study was 2.36 mm with a maximum of 4 mm with forces as low as 60 g for four maxillary incisors. He found that high-pull headgear placed above the center of resistance of the buccal segments counteracts the tip-back moment, controls the steepening of the occlusal plane, and decreases molar extrusion. Dermaut and DeMunck[11] used a modified Burstone[9] technique to intrude incisors with 25 g per tooth. They were able to obtain 3.6 mm of average intrusion. They found no correlation between the amount or duration of intrusion and the amount of root resorption; however, 2.5 mm of mean root resorption did occur. Reitan,[12] in 1974, studied root resorption of human premolar teeth subject to a variety of orthodontic forces. These teeth were later extracted and examined. Although force duration was less than one month, he found that root resorption occurred more frequently in teeth intruded with higher forces. Similar results were found in another short-term human study by Stenvik.[13]

ANIMAL STUDIES OF INTRUSION

Dellinger,[14] in 1967, studied premolar intrusion in monkeys and found that root resorption was not related to the amount of intrusion but was directly related to the force magnitude. Woods[4] found that little if any root resorption occurred in baboons when incisors were intruded. He did find significant resorption when these incisors were uprighted.

STABILITY OF DEEP OVERBITE CORRECTION

The results of most studies concerning the stability of overbite correction indicate a decrease in overbite during treatment followed by an increase in overbite after appliance removal. A study by Berg[15] found only 20 percent relapse of overbite correction with a net total of 40 percent overbite correction. Dake and Sinclair[5] noted overbite relapse of 20–40 percent. Simons[16] found that patients with an initially deep overbite had the deepest overbite 10 years postretention and that protrusion of incisors was correlated with overbite relapse.

Studies have also attempted to relate the stability of deep overbite correction to other factors such as extraction pattern. Cole[17] observed that with extraction therapy, the postretention overbite was deeper than in the original malocclusion. Hernandez[18] studied 83 Class II, Division 1 patients out of retention for a minimum of six months and found more overbite relapse in extraction patients. Walter[19] studied 34 nonextraction patients and found a 2.72-mm overbite decrease with a posttreatment relapse of 0.71 mm. Simons[16] found that postretention relapse was not related to whether or not extractions were performed. Reidel[20] stated that an upright incisor with a large interincisal angle was more likely to relapse. Simons[16] believed that occlusal plane changes during treatment tended to relapse to their original angulation, and this correlated with deep bite relapse. He concluded that mandibular growth, with a vertical component, was correlated with overbite stability.

Overbite may be corrected by extrusion of posterior teeth or intrusion of incisors. Most studies evaluating overbite stability are those in which the overbite was corrected by molar extrusion. Schudy[21] stated that the lower incisors have a very strong tendency to extrude in the posttreatment period and should never be intruded unless unavoidable. Creekmore[22] and Zingeser[23] also reported that incisors should not be intruded except in rare circumstances in which no vertical growth is occurring. This is because molar extrusion to correct deep overbite in patients with no vertical growth is difficult and unstable. The conclusion by Schudy,[21] Creekmore,[22] and Zingeser[23] that intruded incisors relapse was based largely on anecdotal observations. Several recent studies have shown that overbite reduction is achieved primarily by molar extrusion rather than by incisor intrusion.[24–28] Carter[25] and Grano[26] also noted relapse of extruded molars after active treatment even though the patients in Carter's study were still growing.

The only study of the stability of incisor intrusion was done by Dake and Sinclair.[5] They studied incisor intrusion with the utility arch in 30

Class II patients with an overbite of more than 50 percent. All of these patients were treated without extraction while they were still growing. They found that after treatment, maxillary incisors uprighted and extruded about 2 mm after being intruded an average of only 1.2 mm. Since all measurements were made at the incisal edge, it is questionable if true intrusion was achieved or just flaring and molar extrusion. However, deep overbite was successfully treated in these patients since molar extrusion and growth did occur during and following treatment. Dake and Sinclair[5] also stated that lower incisor intrusion during treatment was not associated with posttreatment overbite relapse. The Dake[5] study also noted overbite relapse of 20 percent using reverse curve of Spee wire mechanics and overbite relapse of 34 percent in the group treated with utility arch mechanics.

The literature does not clearly evaluate the stability of deep overbite correction achieved by using anterior intrusive mechanics. This chapter seeks to quantify and evaluate the stability of deep overbite correction using intrusive mechanics in the maxillary arch.

MATERIALS AND METHODS

SAMPLE

Twenty-six patients treated in the Department of Orthodontics, School of Dental Medicine, at the University of Connecticut were used in this study. The mean chronological age of patients at the start of treatment was 14 years. There were 9 males and 17 females in the sample. The mean treatment time was 2.32 years, and the mean posttreatment observation period was two years. Tables 4–1 and 4–2 describe the characteristics of the sample group.

TABLE 4–1   Characteristics of Sample

Variables	Number	Percentage
Males	9	34.6
Females	17	65.4
Extraction Pattern		
Nonextraction	16	61.5
Four bicuspid extraction	5	19.2
Two upper bicuspid exo.	5	19.2
Sex by Extraction Pattern		
Males nonextraction	6	23.1
Males upper bicuspid exo.	0	0
Males four bicuspid exo.	3	11.5
Females nonextraction	10	38.5
Females upper bicuspid exo.	5	19.2
Females four bicuspid exo.	2	7.7

TABLE 4–2   Characteristics of Sample

Variables	T1 Mean	SD	T2 Mean	SD	T3 Mean	SD
Chronologic age (years)	13.96	5.84	16.29	6.02	18.28	6.16
Skeletal age (years)	14.06	5.86	16.39	6.02	18.38	6.12
⊥ to H angle (degrees)*	105.65	8.61	109.19	6.82	109.73	6.71
Interincisal angle (degrees)	134.03	10.56	126.90	10.53	125.02	9.35
Overbite (mm)	5.77	1.33	2.27	0.95	3.07	1.16

Mean treatment time (T1 – T2) = 2.32 years ± 0.89 years.
Mean posttreatment observation period (T2 – T3) = 2 years ± 1.22 years with a range of 0.83–6.75 years.
*Maxillary incisor to H-axis angle (angle 3 of Fig. 4–2).

All patients were treated with the intrusion base arch[9] (Fig. 4–1) in the maxillary arch during the initial phase of treatment. In extraction patients, intrusion was maintained during retraction of incisors with the help of differential moments placed in the archwires. During the finishing phase of treatment, as well as throughout the entire treatment period, no extrusive forces were applied to the maxillary incisors. Most patients were given high-pull headgear to the molars to help control the vertical dimension. Retention consisted of removable maxillary retainers, and all patients were out of active treatment for a minimum of one year. All patients had a lateral cephalometric radiograph taken before treatment (T1), at appliance removal (T2), and at the follow-up retention exam (T3). The control sample was obtained by using the data collected in the Denver Growth Study.[29]

MECHANISM OF INTRUSION

Maxillary incisor intrusion mechanics were comprised of a base arch,[9] posterior anchorage segments joined by a transpalatal arch, and an anterior segment. The posterior anchorage segment is fabricated from rectangular stainless steel wire passively placed in the brackets. Inclusion of second molars in the posterior segment minimizes side effects. A rigid anterior segment on the teeth to be intruded is also placed. The base arch is constructed from .017 × .025 TMA* wire (or a .016 × .022 stainless steel wire with helices mesial to the molar tubes) inserted into the molar auxiliary tube and stepped around the cuspid. The intrusion arch (Fig. 4–1) is not placed directly into the bracket slots of the teeth to be intruded. Inserting the base arch into the slots introduces torque into the

*Ormco Corporation, Glendora, California.

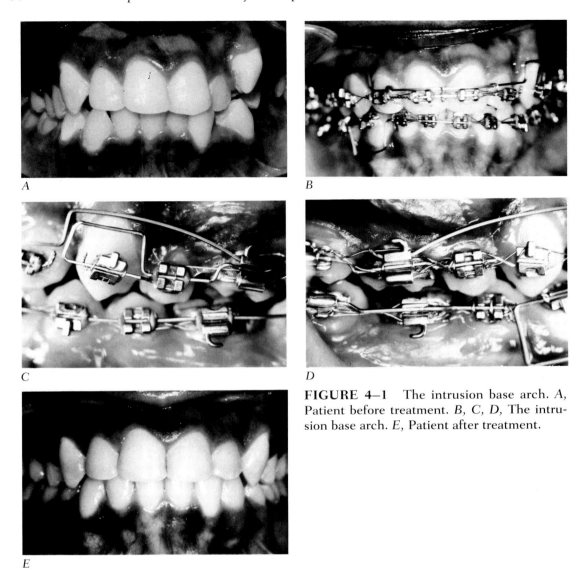

FIGURE 4–1   The intrusion base arch. *A,* Patient before treatment. *B, C, D,* The intrusion base arch. *E,* Patient after treatment.

anterior teeth at placement or as the wire deactivates. If labial root torque were present it would increase the intrusive force and increase side effects on the anchorage unit. Conversely, if lingual root torque were present it would decrease the intrusive force and could actually extrude the anterior teeth.

The base arch is tied to the anterior segment as a point contact. An advantage of ligating the intrusion arch to the anterior segment as a point contact and not into the slots is that the force system is statically determinant, and the amount of intrusive force being delivered can be measured. The intrusion arch is also tied back posteriorly with tension, preferably by steel ligature wires tied to TMA welded stops or to the steel helices. Since the intrusive force is applied anterior to the center of resistance of the

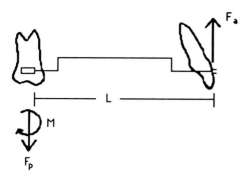

FIGURE 4–2 Force system from an intrusion arch. L, interbracket distance; F_a anterior intrusive force; F_p posterior extrusive force; M, moment that tips posterior segments crown-distal.

$$F_p = F_a$$

$$M = F_a \times Lx$$

anterior segment, this tieback prevents flaring of the anterior teeth.[9] Figure 4–2 shows the force system developed from an activated intrusion arch.

The force levels used for intrusion are important in order to reduce side effects. Side effects of intrusion that can be minimized by using the lowest effective intrusive force possible are (1) posterior extrusion ($F_p = F_a$), (2) buccal segment crown tip-back ($M = F_a \times L$), (3) steepening of the occlusal plane, and (4) apical root resorption. Intrusion forces in this study ranged from approximately 15 to 25 g per tooth. During the subsequent phases of treatment, extrusive forces to the incisors were avoided in order to maintain the achieved intrusion.

METHODOLOGY

Three lateral cephalometric films were traced on acetate paper for each patient. A coordinate system with origin at sella was established on the original head film (T1) of each patient (Fig. 4–3). All measurements were made with reference to this coordinate system. The horizontal (H-axis) was constructed 7° down from the nasion-sella line (NS) to represent the postural horizontal (constructed Frankfort horizontal). Separate maxillary tracings were made transferring the original coordinate system of each patient to this tracing. All measurements were made using an electronic measuring device accurate to the second decimal place. Table 4–3 lists all the variables measured in this study. Treatment changes were calculated by subtracting the value at T2 from T1. Posttreatment changes during retention were calculated by subtracting the value at T3 from T2. Intrusion or superior movement of a point during a time interval is thus assigned a negative value, while extrusion or inferior movement is assigned a positive value.

Superimpositions were made at anterior cranial base structures, and separate maxillary tracings superimposed using the key ridge, lacrimal duct, inferior orbital rim, and palatal contour. The normal eruption of the

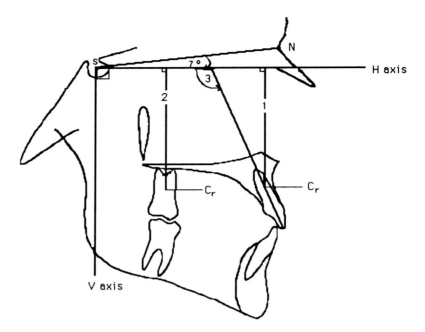

FIGURE 4–3   Coordinate system used for measurements. 1, perpendicular distance of centroid of upper incisor to H-axis; 2, perpendicular distance of centroid of upper molar to H-axis; 3, Angle of long axis of upper incisor to the H-axis.

teeth due to growth was subtracted from the measurements by determining the vertical changes of the maxilla (at the anterior nasal spine[ANS]) and mandible (at menton) at each of the three time periods. Normal growth data obtained from the control group[29] indicated the amount of incisor eruption as a proportion of the change in the vertical dimension measured from ANS to menton. This allowed calculation of the changes in tooth position independent of the effects of normal growth upon the eruption of the teeth.

TABLE 4–3   Variables Measured

 1. Chronologic age.
 2. Skeletal age determined by a hand-wrist radiograph at T1.
 3. Centroid of maxillary incisor to H-axis perpendicular to the H-axis.
 4. Centroid of incisor to H-axis perpendicular to H-axis corrected with growth.
 5. Maxillary incisal edge to H-axis perpendicular to the H-axis.
 6. Incisal edge to H-axis perpendicular to H-axis corrected with growth.
 7. Maxillary incisor long axis to H-axis angle.
 8. Interincisal angle.
 9. Molar centroid to H-axis perpendicular to the H-axis.
10. Molar centroid to H-axis perpendicular to the H-axis corrected with growth.
11. Overbite perpendicular to the H-axis.
12. ANS to menton distance perpendicular to the H-axis.

The centroid for the anterior segment was estimated using average central incisor root and crown lengths. The estimated anterior centroid is a point 3/10 of the root length from the cemento-enamel junction along the long axis of the tooth.[30] Since the root apex and cemento-enamel junction are difficult to determine on lateral cephalometric films, the incisal edge of the central was used as the origin to detect the centroid. The centroid was calculated to be 17 mm from the incisal edge of the central incisor along its long axis.[10] This measurement was made on all films by indexing the incisor template used for tracing. Although the centroid is not a true center of rotation or center of resistance, it was a constant estimate throughout the study. The centroid was used because any tipping that occurs will not significantly affect the horizontal and vertical position of the centroid, since this is the estimated point about which the tooth rotates. It should be noted that the incisal edge or root apex is not used because any tipping will significantly affect the horizontal and vertical positions of these points. By using the centroid, the amount of incisor intrusion and relapse was determined because rotation of the central incisor has little effect on the measured amount of intrusion relative to the centroid.[10]

To measure the amount of extrusion of the posterior segment, a posterior centroid was used. This was estimated to be at the furcation of the first molar.[31] This point was estimated and indexed on the molar template and was held constant throughout the study.

RESULTS

Tables 4–4 through 4–8 show the overbite changes and the changes in tooth position as measured from cranial base and maxillary superimpositions. Overbite (Table 4–4) showed a mean reduction of 3.31 mm (57.36 percent) during treatment, and a mean relapse of 0.80 mm (24.17 percent) was observed during the posttreatment period. The mean overall reduction in overbite from T1 to T3 was 43.5 percent. The overall change in overbite from T1 to T3 showed a statistically significant difference ($p < 0.001$) when a paired t-test was performed.

Changes in the vertical dimension, as measured from ANS to menton, were assessed to determine if overbite correction increased the vertical dimension with respect to the control group by hinging the mandible open. Incremental growth data were used as the control. During treatment the increase in the vertical dimension (Table 4–8) showed a distribution similar to that during the posttreatment period. Overbite stability and relapse did not show significant correlation ($p < 0.05$) with the vertical growth changes. Furthermore, the occurrence of vertical growth did not correlate with any of the variables measured (Table 4–3).

Table 4–7 shows that after taking normal eruption into consideration, the maxillary incisors were intruded an average of 2.32 mm ($p < 0.0001$)

TABLE 4–4   Treatment and Posttreatment Vertical Changes from Cranial Base Superimpositions. All Measurements Are Made Perpendicular to the H-Axis.

Variables	Treatment Change		Posttreatment Change	
	mm[a]	SD	mm[a]	SD
Maxillary incisor centroid to H-axis	+0.42	1.75 ns	+1.01	1.19***
Maxillary incisal edge to H-axis	+0.50	1.86 ns	+1.08	1.10****
Maxillary incisor to H-axis angle (degrees)	+3.54	8.19*	+0.54	3.70 ns
Interincisal angle (degrees)	−4.81	13.86**	−0.35	7.15 ns
Maxillary molar centroid to H-axis	+1.69	1.79***	+0.43	0.76**
Overbite	−3.31	1.42****	+0.80	0.80****
Vertical dimension (ANS to menton)	+3.25	2.80	+0.75	1.22

[a] (−) indicates intrusion occurred or a decrease in the measurement occurred; (+) indicates extrusion occurred or an increase in the measurement occurred.
ns: not a statistically significant change.
*Statistically significant change: $p < 0.05$.
**Statistically significant change: $p < 0.01$.
***Statistically significant change: $p < 0.001$.
****Statistically significant change: $p < 0.0001$.

TABLE 4–5   Treatment and Posttreatment Vertical Changes from Cranial Base Superimpositions Mathematically Eliminating the Effect of Growth upon the Eruption of the Teeth. All Measurements Are Made Perpendicular to the H-Axis and Indicate the Actual Changes in Tooth Position.

Variables	Treatment Change		Posttreatment Change	
	mm[a]	SD	mm[a]	SD
Maxillary incisor centroid to H-axis	−0.87	1.33**	+0.69	1.02**
Maxillary incisal edge to H-axis	−0.78	1.35**	+0.79	0.88***
Maxillary molar centroid to H-axis	+1.69	1.79***	+0.43	0.76**

[a] (−) indicates intrusion occurred or a decrease in the measurement occurred; (+) indicates extrusion occurred or an increase in the measurement occurred.
*Statistically significant change: $p < 0.05$.
**Statistically significant change: $p < 0.01$.
***Statistically significant change: $p < 0.001$.
****Statistically significant change: $p < 0.0001$.

TABLE 4–6   Treatment and Posttreatment Vertical Changes from Maxillary Superimpositions. All Measurements Are Made Perpendicular to the H-Axis.

Variables	Treatment Change		Posttreatment Change	
	mm[a]	SD	mm[a]	SD
Maxillary incisor centroid to H-axis	−1.08	0.75****	+0.40	0.14**
Maxillary incisal edge to H-axis	−1.15	0.74****	+0.42	0.62**
Maxillary molar centroid to H-axis	+1.38	1.26****	+0.13	0.44 ns

[a] (−) indicates intrusion occurred or a decrease in the measurement occurred; (+) indicates extrusion occurred or an increase in the measurement occurred.
ns: not a statistically significant change.
*Statistically significant change: $p < 0.05$.
**Statistically significant change: $p < 0.01$.
***Statistically significant change: $p < 0.001$.
****Statistically significant change: $p < 0.0001$.

during treatment. Relapse of the intrusion during T2 to T3 was only 0.15 mm, a statistically insignificant change. Table 4–7 also shows that the maxillary molar was only negligibly extruded (0.03 mm) during treatment due to the anterior intrusive mechanics. This was a statistically and clinically insignificant change.

The interincisal angle and the inclination of the maxillary incisor as related to the H-axis were evaluated at T2 and T3 to determine if the patients were finished with clinically acceptable axial inclinations of the teeth (Table 4–8). Almost all angles at T2 and T3 were within 2 standard deviations of the normal values.[29] The interincisal angle and the upper incisor to H-axis angle did not show statistically significant changes during the posttreatment period.

Analysis of variance was performed to determine if there were any differences between the nonextraction, two-upper-bicuspid extraction, and four-bicuspid extraction groups. No differences were found except that the extraction groups had more intrusion than the nonextraction group (Tables 4–6 and 4–7).

TABLE 4–7 Treatment and Posttreatment Vertical Changes from Maxillary Superimpositions Mathematically Eliminating the Effect of Growth upon the Eruption of the Teeth. All Measurements Are Made Perpendicular to the H-Axis and Indicate the Actual Changes in Tooth Position.

	Treatment Change		Posttreatment Change	
Variables	*mm[a]*	*SD*	*mm[a]*	*SD*
Maxillary incisor centroid to H-axis	−2.32	1.33****	+0.15	0.55 ns
Maxillary incisal edge to H-axis	−2.07	1.62****	+0.13	0.61 ns
Maxillary molar centroid to H-axis	+0.03	1.22 ns	−0.15	0.51 ns

[a] (−) indicates intrusion occurred or a decrease in the measurement occurred; (+) indicates extrusion occurred or an increase in the measurement occurred.
ns: not a statistically significant change.
*Statistically significant change: $p < 0.05$.
**Statistically significant change: $p < 0.01$.
***Statistically significant change: $p < 0.001$.
****Statistically significant change: $p < 0.0001$.

TABLE 4–8 Description of Z-scores and Their Distribution

Variable	*Mean Z-score*	*Skewness of Z-score*	*Standard Error of Skewness*
ANS–menton treatment change	2.28	4.11	0.46
ANS–menton posttreatment change	2.59	4.62	0.46
Maxillary incisor to H-axis angle at T2	0.76	0.66	0.46
Maxillary incisor to H-axis angle at T3	0.72	0.81	0.46
Interincisal angle at T2	0.95	0.85	0.46
Interincisal angle at T3	0.91	0.54	0.46

Skewness = $\dfrac{\sum (x - \bar{x})^3}{n - 1}$

Standard error of skewness = square root of $6/n$.

Analysis of variance was also performed to determine if there were any significant differences in measurements between the sexes. More incisor intrusion was seen in females as measured from cranial base superimpositions (Table 4–4) from both the centroid and the incisal edge. On the other hand, males showed more molar extrusion and more overbite correction during treatment (3.77 mm for males and 3.06 mm for females). Contrary to cranial base superimpositions, maxillary superimpositions (Table 4–7) for males showed more incisor intrusion (3.39 mm) than females (1.74 mm) when measured from the centroid. The difference in the results from the two superimpositions is explained by males showing significantly more growth ($p < 0.01$) in the vertical dimension as measured from ANS to menton during treatment (Table 4–4). Males had a mean increase of 5.49 mm at ANS to menton during treatment while females had 2.14 mm.

Correlations were calculated for all variables at all the time intervals. Overbite relapse correlated with the amount of overbite correction. The more the overbite was corrected during treatment, the more it tended to relapse during the period T2 to T3. Overbite relapse also correlated with both incisor intrusion relapse measured from the centroid and incisal edge and with molar posttreatment change (Table 4–7). The more the maxillary incisor extruded (or the maxillary molar intruded) during T2 to T3, the more the overbite increased during this period.

Figure 4–4 shows tracings of patient J. S., a 14-year-old female treated without extraction. During the 2.6 years of treatment minimal growth occurred, and overbite was mostly corrected by upper incisor intrusion. During the posttreatment period of 1.5 years no vertical growth occurred, and only slight incisor extrusion occurred.

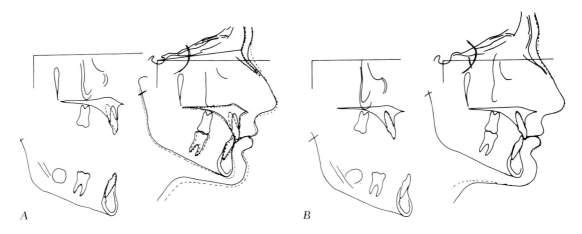

FIGURE 4–4   Superimpositions of patient J. S. *A*, Treatment changes. The solid line represents initial tracing (T1) and the broken line represents deband tracing (T2). *B*, Posttreatment changes. The solid line represents deband tracing (T2) and the broken line represents final tracing (T3).

Figure 4–5 shows tracings of patient G. C., a 14.3-year-old male treated with extraction of four first bicuspids. The overbite was corrected primarily by upper incisor intrusion. The upper molar was not extruded as it was moved into the extraction site. During the 4.4-year posttreatment period, the lower incisor flared slightly, and the upper incisor position was stable.

Figure 4–6 shows tracings of patient R. N., an 11.2-year-old female treated without extraction. During the 2.25-year treatment period significant growth occurred. During the 1.1-year posttreatment period minimal growth and no relapse in the maxilla were seen.

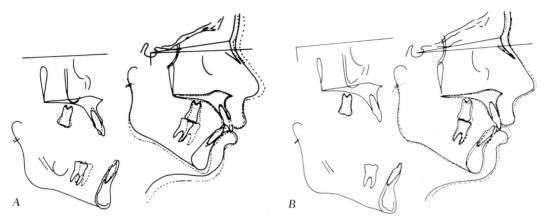

FIGURE 4–5   Superimpositions of patient G. C. *A,* Treatment changes. The solid line represents initial tracing (T1) and the broken line represents deband tracing (T2). *B,* Posttreatment changes. The solid line represents deband tracing (T2) and the broken line represents final tracing (T3).

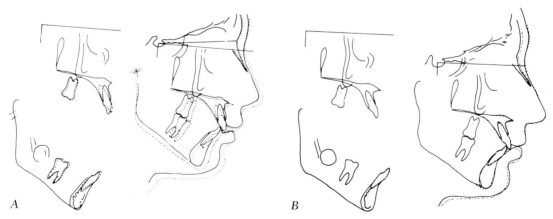

FIGURE 4–6.   Superimpositions of patient R. N. *A,* Treatment changes. The solid line represents initial tracing (T1) and the broken line represents deband tracing (T2). *B,* Posttreatment changes. The solid line represents deband tracing (T2) and the broken line represents final tracing (T3).

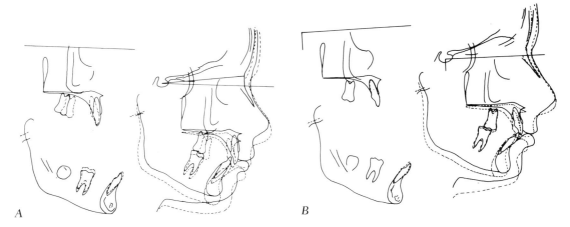

A   B

FIGURE 4–7   Superimpositions of patient E. P. *A,* Treatment changes. The solid line represents initial tracing (T1) and the broken line represents deband tracing (T2). *B,* Posttreatment changes. The solid line represents deband tracing (T2) and the broken line represents final tracing (T3).

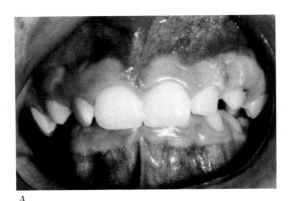

A

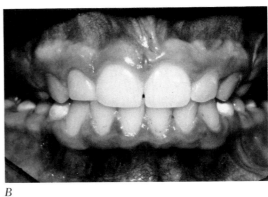

B

FIGURE 4–8   Patient treated with intrusive mechanics. *A,* Before treatment (T1). *B,* At deband (T2). *C,* Two years posttreatment (T3).

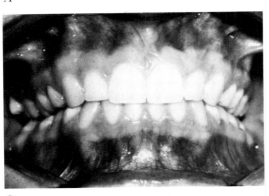

C

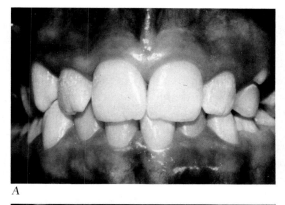

A

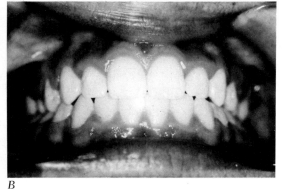

B

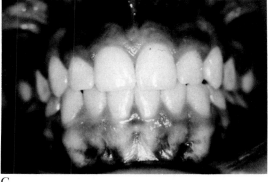

C

FIGURE 4–9   Patient treated with intrusive mechanics. *A,* Before treatment (T1). *B,* At deband (T2). *C,* Two years posttreatment (T3).

Figure 4–7 shows tracings of patient E. P., an 11.5-year-old female treated with upper bicuspid extractions. During the treatment period this patient showed a large amount of growth as both the maxilla and mandible moved inferiorly. During the 6.7-year posttreatment period significant growth occurred, but the tooth positions remained fairly stable.

Figure 4–8A shows a patient with over 100 percent overbite at the start of treatment. With the intrusion base arch the overbite is reduced to normal at the end of treatment (Fig. 4–8B). Two years posttreatment (Fig. 4–8C) there is only a slight increase in the overbite. Figure 4–9 shows another patient treated with intrusive mechanics. In this patient the result (Fig. 4–9C) is very stable.

DISCUSSION

Deep overbite can be corrected by intrusion of incisors and some extrusion of molars and by allowing favorable vertical growth to occur. In the present study, the deep overbite was primarily corrected by genuine incisor intrusion. The maxillary molar did not significantly extrude/erupt during treatment when compared to the control group. This prevented the mandible from being iatrogenically hinged open during treatment.

Björk,[32] Pearson,[33,34] and Burstone[35] have stressed that a counterclockwise (forward) mandibular rotation is desirable in patients with a long lower facial height or with a steep mandibular plane angle (high-angle patients). To achieve these objectives it is important to prevent molar extrusive mechanics and to control passive eruption of molars into the interocclusal space, especially in growing patients. Treatment planning of deep-overbite correction should consider the growth potential of the patient as well as the vertical skeletal pattern. In the present study, many of the patients had adverse vertical characteristics that prompted the correction of deep overbite by using anterior intrusive mechanics. Extrusive mechanics would have caused a significant hinging open of the mandible, resulting in an increase in the lower facial height, a steepening of the occlusal plane, and an increase in the interlabial gap.

In some patients the mandible rotated clockwise (open) due to the patients' normal growth pattern. This growth effect contributed to some of the overbite correction observed during treatment. This normal molar extrusion/eruption occurring with vertical growth aided in the overbite correction seen during treatment. Hemley,[1] Strang,[2] and Sleichter[3] have described that deep overbite can be successfully corrected by molar extrusion in growing patients. The present study illustrates that deep overbite correction by intrusion minimizes the contribution of molar extrusion in the overall treatment of deep bite.

Since the lower vertical facial height (ANS to menton) changes during treatment were similar to the changes during the posttreatment period, the intrusive mechanics did not alter the patients' growth pattern during treatment. This also indicates that during treatment there was good control of the vertical dimension and vertical position of the maxillary molar.

The present study showed that 2.32 mm of average maxillary incisor intrusion was possible. The minimum intrusion obtained was 0.31 mm with a maximum of 4.82 mm of maxillary incisor intrusion. Studies by Dake and Sinclair,[5] Otto,[8] and Greig[7] showed that similar amounts of lower incisor intrusion are possible, but these studies measured intrusion from the incisal edge and not from a centroid. These studies also used samples that were still growing and did not attempt to account for the normal eruption of the teeth that occurs with vertical facial growth. The study by Gottlieb[10] showed that up to 4 mm of incisor intrusion was possible, but Gottlieb's study was performed during a short time interval so that growth was not a factor. The present study suggests that overbite correction by intrusion would be stable in a nongrowing sample, since true incisor intrusion appears to be stable when growth effects upon the eruption of teeth are mathematically eliminated.

In the present study, overbite was reduced 3.31 mm during treatment. Although the 0.8 mm of overbite relapse was statistically significant ($p < 0.0001$), this posttreatment change may not be clinically relevant (Figs. 4–8 and 4–9). This amounts to a 24.17 percent mean overbite posttreatment change, which is similar to that noted in other studies by Sinclair,[5] Berg,[15] and Simons.[16] A study by Glenn[36] also found overbite to be stable during the postretention period. In the present study, the mean overbite at the end of treatment was 2.27 mm, and this increased to 3.1 mm at the end of the posttreatment period. This suggests that overcorrection of a deep bite at the end of treatment might be a desirable goal. Although deep-bite correction with intrusive mechanics has posttreatment overbite changes similar to those with other mechanics,[5,15,16] intrusion has the clear advantage of providing better control of the vertical dimension, as explained earlier.

The intrusion of the maxillary incisors was stable, since only 0.15 mm of posttreatment extrusion occurred. This contradicts Schudy[21] who, in 1968, suggested that incisor intrusion is not stable. The present study shows that the maxillary incisor intrusion relapse accounted for only 0.15 mm of the total 0.80 mm of overbite relapse. This finding is also significant considering that 2.32 mm of this correction was due to maxillary incisor intrusion.

The results indicate that the more the overbite was corrected, the more it tended to relapse during the posttreatment period. Overbite relapse during the posttreatment period was positively correlated with incisor extrusion and molar changes during the posttreatment period. Overbite relapse, however, did not correlate with the amount of molar extrusion during treatment, possibly because there was minimal molar extrusion during treatment. The stability of molar extrusion in growing patients was examined in several previous studies[24-28] which suggest that this method of overbite correction was fairly stable when the interocclusal space was not violated.

It is believed that the interincisal angle may play a critical role in the stability of deep overbite correction. Reidel[20] suggests that a large interincisal angle at the end of treatment may relate to the relapse of deep overbite. Reidel showed that an upright incisor at the end of treatment may also relate to deep overbite relapse. In the present study, the incisor axial inclinations and overbite did not significantly change during the posttreatment period. This suggests that good axial inclinations of the teeth at the end of treatment may be a factor in the stability of the final result, as Reidel suggests.[20]

Extraction pattern has been suggested as playing a role in the stability of deep overbite correction.[16-19] The present study found no difference in stability between the extraction and nonextraction groups, supporting the findings of Simons.[16] However, Little[37] found a statistically significant increase in overbite during the postretention period for 65 first bicuspid extraction patients. The increase in overbite in Little's study was only 0.76 mm, which, as stated previously, may not be clinically significant. Although the number of extraction patients in the present study was small, it suggests that deep overbite correction with intrusive mechanics is equally stable in both extraction and nonextraction patients.

REFERENCES

1. Hemley S: Bite plates: Their application and action. Am J Orthod 24:721–736, 1938.
2. Strang RH, Thompson W: Textbook of Orthodontics, 4th ed. Philadelphia, Lea and Febiger, 1958.
3. Sleichter CG: Effects of maxillary bite plane therapy in orthodontics. Am J Orthod 40:850–870, 1954.
4. Woods MG: The mechanics of lower incisor intrusion: Experiments in nongrowing baboons. Am J Orthod 93:186–195, 1988.
5. Dake ML, Sinclair PM: A comparison of the Ricketts and Tweed-type arch leveling techniques. Am J Orthod 95:72–78, 1989.
6. Ricketts RW: Bioprogressive therapy. Rocky Mountain Orthod. Denver, CO, 1979.
7. Greig DGM: Bioprogressive therapy: Overbite reduction with the lower utility arch. Br J Orthod 10:214–216, 1983.
8. Otto RL, Anholm JM, Engle GA: A comparative analysis of intrusion of incisor teeth achieved in adults and children according to facial type. Am J Orthod 77:437–446, 1980.
9. Burstone CJ: Deep overbite correction by intrusion. Am J Orthod 72:1–22, 1977.
10. Gottlieb BS: The effects of an intrusive base arch on tooth position: A radiographic study. Thesis, University of Connecticut, 1979.
11. Dermaut LR, DeMunck A: Apical root resorption of upper incisors caused by intrusive tooth movement: A radiographic study. Am J Orthod 90:321–329, 1986.
12. Reitan K: Initial tissue behavior during apical root resorption. Angle Orthod 44:68–82, 1974.
13. Stenvik A, Mjor IA: Pulp and dentine reactions to experimental tooth intrusion. Am J Orthod 57:370–385, 1970.
14. Dellinger EL: A histological and cephalometric investigation of premolar intrusion in the Macaca speciosa monkey. Am J Orthod 53:325–355, 1967.
15. Berg R: Stability of deep overbite correction. European J Orthod 5:75–83, 1983.
16. Simons ME, Joondeph DR: Change in overbite: A ten-year post-retention study. Am J Orthod 64:349–367, 1973.
17. Cole HJ: Certain results of extraction in the treatment of malocclusion. Angle Orthod 18:103–113, 1948.
18. Hernandez JL: Mandibular bicanine width relative to overbite. Am J Orthod 56:455–467, 1969.
19. Walter DC: Changes in the form and dimensions of dental arches resulting from orthodontic treatment. Angle Orthod 23:3–18, 1953.
20. Reidel RA: A review of the retention problem. Angle Orthod 30:179–194, 1960.
21. Schudy FF: The control of vertical overbite in clinical orthodontics. Angle Orthod 38:19–39, 1968.
22. Creekmore TD: Inhibition or stimulation of vertical growth of the facial complex. Angle Orthod 37:285–297, 1967.
23. Zingeser MR: Vertical response to class II division 1 therapy. Angle Orthod 34:58–64, 1964.

24. Barton JJ: A cephalometric comparison of cases treated with Edgewise and Begg techniques. Angle Orthod 43:119–126, 1973.

25. Carter NE: First premolar extractions and fixed appliances in class II division 1 malocclusion. British J Orthod 15:1–10, 1988.

26. Grano DJ: A radiographic cephalometric study of certain tooth movements observed in the post-retention period of deep overbite cases treated with the Begg technique. Am J Orthod 60:202–203, 1971.

27. Menezes DM: Changes in tooth position and vertical dimension in severe class II division 1 cases during Begg treatment. British J Orthod 2:85–91, 1975.

28. O'Reilly MT: Treatment and post-treatment changes with the Begg appliance. Am J Orthod 75:535–547, 1879.

29. Burstone CJ, Hickman J: University of Connecticut Health Center Monograph. Denver Growth Study Data, 1968.

30. Burstone CJ: Holographic determination of centers of rotation produced by orthodontic forces. Am J Orthod 77:396, 1980.

31. Dermaut LR, Kleutghen JJ, DeClerck HH: Experimental determination of the center of resistance of the upper first molar in a macerated, dry human skull submitted to horizontal headgear traction. Am J Orthod 90:29–36, 1986.

32. Björk A. Prediction of mandibular growth rotation. Am J Orthod 55:585–599, 1969.

33. Pearson LE: Vertical control in treatment of patients having backward rotational growth tendencies. Angle Orthod 48:132–140, 1978.

34. Pearson LE: Vertical control in fully banded orthodontic treatment. Angle Orthod 56:205–224, 1986.

35. Burstone CJ: Lip posture and its significance in treatment planning. Am J Orthod 53:262–284, 1967.

36. Glenn G, Sinclair P, Alexander R: Nonextraction orthodontic therapy; Post-treatment dental and skeletal stability. Am J Orthod 92:321–328, 1987.

37. Little R, Riedel R, Wallen T: Stability and relapse of mandibular anterior alignment—First premolar extraction cases treated by traditional edgewise orthodontics. Am J Orthod 80:349–365.

The Effects of Premolar Extractions on the Long-Term Stability of the Mandibular Incisors

John C. Gorman

The controversy regarding the role of extractions in preventing relapse of orthodontic treatment still exists after nearly a century of debate. The most recent studies seem to indicate that extraction is not a panacea and that long-term stability of lower incisor correction can be expected in only about 20 percent of extraction cases. Other studies are not so pessimistic and suggest that treatment techniques and retention plans may be major factors in long-term stability.

"Twelve Keys to Stability," developed after 28 years of clinical practice, are given here, and a description of individualized retention plans is presented.

The role of premolar extraction in orthodontics has been fiercely debated since the turn of the century. Angle, Case, Dewey, Tweed, Ricketts, Begg, and Cetlin have each guided the pendulum of our "professional clock."

At the most recent meeting of the Great Lakes Association of Orthodontists, two incidents indicated to me just how far the pendulum has swung in favor of nonextraction treatment since the 1960s when it stood at the outer limits in favor of extraction.

First, one of the principal speakers at the meeting stated that his goal in treating children was to "keep his extraction rate below 20 percent." By initiating treatment early, he was able to achieve good occlusions even in severely crowded cases. Intraoral photographs demonstrated considerable expansion and change in arch form during treatment.

The second incident involved a discussion with a graduate student from one of our most respected universities. He was displaying a a series of cases treated at his school, most of which were expanded during treatment. In discussing long-term stability with this student, his response to why teeth had not been removed in several cases was, "It's common knowledge that it makes no difference whether you extract or not. All cases collapse after retention is removed, so why extract?"

My orthodontic training at Washington University in the early sixties was predominately nonextraction, utilizing the twin wire and labial-lingual appliances. The difficulty in maintaining anterior alignment postretention and the full profiles produced by arch expansion soon led me to the Begg Society where premolar extractions were advised in about 80 percent of our patients. Discouraged by the unattractive faces I was creating by over-retraction of the anterior teeth and the opening of the mandibular plane angle, I looked for another method of treatment.

I finally found an "orthodontic home" at the Tweed Foundation. Anchorage preparation, control of the vertical dimension, upright lower incisors, and an aversion to expansion of any kind required an extraction rate of about 65 percent.

After practicing the Tweed philosophy for 24 years and having had the opportunity to see many former patients 10 or more years after discontinuing all retention, I can make the following empirical observation: Very few patients, whether treated with or without extraction, escape some degree of postretention change. However, the vast majority of my patients whose end-of-treatment records indicate strict adherence to Tweed objectives have lower incisor alignment that is within an acceptable range even after 20 years.

While there appears to be general agreement that extractions are justified in correcting bimaxillary protrusions or severe arch length deficiencies, the debate continues on the role premolar extractions play in the long-term stability of incisor alignment.

In his text *Contemporary Orthodontics*, Proffit[1] states that first premolar teeth are often extracted to allow better lip contours and to provide a more stable result. Yet the most recent studies[2] on relapse of the lower incisors in cases where extraction of premolars was performed indicate a discouraging result might be expected in at least two thirds of patients.

This chapter reviews the existing research and provides some candid observations based on 28 years of clinical practice.

LITERATURE REVIEW

Enlow[3] defined relapse as "a histogenetic and morphogenic response to some anatomical and functional violation of an existing state of anatomic and functional balance." It is usually thought of as a "rebound" movement in which teeth recoil back somewhere close to their original positions once retentive forces are removed. Enlow doesn't accept the idea that the relapse process is merely a passive mechanical recoil reaction of the PDM to stresses placed on its fibers. He states that periodontal fibers have a great capacity for remodeling and can accommodate virtually any tooth position if a regional state of anatomic and physiologic balance exists.

Over 200 articles have been published in the last 50 years dealing with orthodontic relapse. Early writings stressed the importance of placing the teeth in excellent occlusion and holding them there until the perioral musculature adapted to their new positions. Lower incisor crowding that developed postretention was attributed to a failure of the muscles to adapt.

Angle's[4] statement in 1907 that "The problem involved in retention is so great as to test the utmost skill of the most competent orthodontist, often being greater than the difficulties being encountered in the treatment of the case up to this point" appears to be as true today as it was then.

Mershon[5] stated that the final position of the teeth was like "an argument with Mother Nature," who always won.

Hawley[6] said that he would "give half his fee to anyone who would be responsible for the retention of his results when the active appliance was removed."

Begg[7] attributed crowding to the lack of attrition interproximally due to the diet of modern man and advocated extractions to prevent this from occurring.

Tweed,[8] one of Angle's most ardent supporters, was so discouraged by postretention relapse that he seriously considered giving up the profession. He examined 70 percent of the patients he had treated after six and a half years of orthodontic practice following Angle's philosophy that demanded a full complement of teeth. To his amazement he found that only 20 percent of the cases met his orthodontic objectives, which were:

1 Stability of end result—teeth that remain in their corrected position.

2. Healthy investing tissues, ensuring longevity of the denture.

3. A dental apparatus that can do its work efficiently.

4. The best in facial aesthetics.

Following this humbling experience, Tweed began treatment of similar bimaxillary protrusion cases, half by "conventional" nonextraction treatment and half by the removal of four first premolars.

In the first group he reported mesial displacement of the incisors from their normal positions and a resultant collapse of the mandibular arch in the incisal region.

In the second group, where four premolars had been extracted and the mandibular incisors correctly positioned with relation to basal bone, the cases remained free from serious relapse following one year of retention. Retreatment of the patients whose dentures were left in bimaxillary protrusion after removal of four premolars resulted in similar stability several years postretention.

In his text *Clinical Orthodontics*, published 22 years after he reported the results of his extraction experiment, Tweed[9] stated that determining the anterior limits of the denture was the key to stability. He said that whenever he was able to comply with the requirements of the diagnostic facial triangle, retention problems were of little concern in his practice.

In an interview in 1968, Tweed[10] reported that in patients who exhibited a class C growth trend, where mandibular growth exceeds maxillary growth in a downward and forward direction, there was more likelihood of lower incisor relapse. Since Tweed felt that 75 percent of his patients followed a type C growth trend, he recommended placing a fixed cuspid-to-cuspid retainer in the mandibular arch and leaving it there until growth was complete. In those few patients who presented retention problems he felt that abnormal muscle function was the principle cause of relapse.

As a student of Tweed's, and later as an instructor at the Tweed Foundation, I recall very little time being spent on teaching retention. The premise was, and still is, that if a case is properly diagnosed and treated to Tweed standards, postretention relapse will be minimal.

The validity of this premise is certainly not universally accepted, and in light of the conflicting results of many studies on postretention stability it is often totally disregarded.

Studies by Little and others[2,11–16] at the University of Washington concluded that extraction of premolar teeth has little effect on long-term (10–20 years) posttreatment stability of lower incisor alignment. The cases studied were collected from the orthodontic clinic at the University of Washington and from practices of the faculty. Class I and Class II cases were included in each study. Significant data reported in seven published articles point to several conclusions:

1. Arch length decreases postretention.

2. Intercanine width decreases postretention.

3. Overbite deepens postretention.

4. Neither age, sex, Angle classification, growth, nor extraction has any effect on the stability of orthodontically rotated teeth postretention.

5. The more severely a tooth is rotated pretreatment, the greater its tendency to relapse postretention.

6. Only 30 percent of the premolar extraction cases in this sample had satisfactory alignment of the lower incisors 10 years postretention, and only 10 percent exhibited good alignment 20 years postretention.

7. Untreated orthodontic normals showed a decrease in arch length, a decrease in intercanine width, and lower incisor irregularity, but to a lesser degree than treated cases.

8. Long-term response to mandibular alignment is unpredictable, with no apparent predictors of future success when considering pretreatment records or the treated results.

9. Cases that exhibit mandibular spacing before treatment continue to lose arch length postretention. Spaces do not reappear, and crowding can occur.

Some of these conclusions, such as arch length decrease, intercanine width decrease, and overbite deepening, have been reached by other investigators.[17–19] However, studies of different populations have produced results with a much greater incidence of mandibular incisor stability.

Sadowsky[20] reported on the stability of 96 cases examined an average of 20 years after retention. Patients were treated by five Chicago area practitioners. These patients all exhibited "100 percent correction" of the lower incisor crowding present at the initiation of treatment. A comparison of the long-term result to the original malocclusion showed there was increased mandibular crowding in 9 percent of the cases. At the long-term follow-up, 15 percent of the cases had crowding beyond 3 mm, and only 1 percent had crowding of 6.5 mm or more. It should be pointed out that Sadowsky used a different method of measuring lower incisor crowding than the University of Washington studies; however, both investigators used a subjective approach to what constituted acceptable incisor alignment. There was no attempt to distinguish between cases treated by the extraction or nonextraction approaches in Sadowsky's study. In a later article by Uhde, Sadowsky, and Begole,[17] the sample was broken down into 45 nonextraction and 27 extraction cases. The extraction sample showed more severe crowding at the beginning of treatment and a smaller percentage of relapse postretention.

Glenn[18] studied 28 cases of nonextraction treatment an average of eight years postretention. All patients were treated by the same orthodontist. He found that incisor irregularity increased slightly postretention. Relapse patterns were similar to, though greater than, those seen in Sinclair's[14] untreated normal population. They were only one half as severe as those seen in Little's[2,12] studies. Lower incisors were proclined during treatment, when measured to the A-PO line, an average of 1.4 mm and tended to remain stable postretention. Class II malocclusions with large ANB differences showed the most lower incisor relapse postretention. The severity of relapse seemed to bear a direct relationship to the severity of the original malocclusion.

Sandusky[21] reported on postretention stability of 85 extraction cases treated by Tweed and Tweed Foundation members. He reported less than 10 percent relapse of the lower incisors using Little's irregularity index. He found the lower incisors tended to move forward postretention and the occlusal plane—Frankfort horizontal plane—angle decreased.

Tweed[10] talked in a 1968 interview about a study he was conducting with 100 extraction and 100 nonextraction cases examined 25 years postretention. While no scientific data are available, Tweed's conclusion was that the extraction cases were more stable.

In a master's degree thesis at Loma Linda, Davis[22] reported that extraction cases experienced less mandibular incisor crowding and were more stable than nonextraction cases three to five years postretention.

Kuftinic and Strom[23] examined 50 cases, 25 extraction and 25 nonextraction, four months or more after discontinuing retention and found that lower incisor relapse was greater in nonextraction cases.

Other studies related to mandibular incisor stability have focused on different concerns. El-Mangoury[24] divided 50 well-treated cases into two groups of 25 each. Group I was stable and Group II had relapsed. He found that the intercanine width decreased twice as much in the relapsed group.

Sharpe[25] examined 10-year posttreatment records of 36 patients and concluded that there may be a relationship between orthodontic relapse and the parameters of increased root resorption and decreased crestal bone levels.

Following the advice of Reitan[26] in his 1969 paper, "Principles of Retention and Avoidance of Posttreatment Relapse," which suggested that relapse of rotated teeth could be minimized by overcorrection or removal of supralveolar structures, Edwards[27] and Boese[28] reported on circumferential fiberotomy.

Edwards[27] performed fiberotomies on 16 teeth and advised that this technique did appear to be a simple method of alleviating much of the relapse problem of rotated teeth.

Boese[28] published a study on 40 extraction cases that were orthodontically treated but never retained. His findings were based on observations made four to nine years posttreatment. All patients had undergone fiberotomy and reproximation of the mandibular incisors. Crowding was evaluated by Little's irregularity index and was found to be almost nonexistent posttreatment. It should be noted that about one half of the cases required more than 1.8 mm of enamel reduction, performed in several stages. It is also interesting to note that the lower incisors were uprighted during treatment and continued to upright posttreatment. The mean values for IMPA (89.5 at appliance removal, 88.6 postretention) are within the range that Tweed suggested was necessary for stability. Those patients whose growth would have been classified as type C by Tweed required additional amounts of reproximation as growth occurred. Slight overcorrection of rotations was accomplished at least six months prior to performing the fiberotomies.

Boese[28] felt that the practice of not utilizing any retention in the mandibular arch played an important role in stabilizing the lower anterior teeth. He stated that "lower retention eliminates the need for reproximation, since it postpones natural arch length loss, prevents any compensatory lower incisor movement, and allows for a build up of forces during the retention period. The decision not to use lower retention will allow for natural arch length loss which occurs gradually and can be dealt with immediately."

DISCUSSION

I have attempted to find some common denominators that might explain the differences between the results of the University of Washington studies and those of other investigators.

Since Sandusky's[21] study showed the greatest degree of stability postretention and Little's[12] studies showed the most relapse, a comparison of their reports was attempted.

In Sandusky's sample, lower incisors appear to have been uprighted more than in Little's sample. There was very little expansion of intercanine width in Sandusky's cases, while 60 percent of the patients in the University of Washington study showed canine expansion of more than 1 mm during treatment.

In the Tweed sample, there was extensive use of tip-back bends and anchorage preparation with Class III elastics. In the Washington sample there was minimal use of these mechanics. From examining the photographs of 30 cases in Little's sample, published in his 1981 article, there appears to have been overcorrection of lower incisor rotations in only two cases, both of which had postretention stability within acceptable limits.

While no photographs were available to examine Sandusky's cases, it is common practice for Tweed orthodontists to overcorrect incisor rotations. Little pointed out that perhaps as many as half of the rotations or displacements in his sample returned in a pattern different from that in the original condition.

Parker[29] stated in his article "Retention—Retainers May Be Forever" that "experience does not give wisdom but it may and should grant perspective."

With over 28 years of orthodontic experience, my perspective on retention has changed from an expectation of universal stability following bicuspid extraction and two years of retention to the realization that individual retention plans must be developed for each patient.

The problem of posttreatment stability of the lower incisors is discussed during the initial consultation. I explain that our treatment fee includes one year of retention visits and that most of our patients require additional retention, for which there is a modest charge. At the posttreatment consultation these points are reemphasized, and our individual plan for retention is outlined. Development of the plan is based on the following assumptions:

1. Arch length will decrease.

2. Intercanine width can be expected to return to the original or less.

3. The amount and direction of posttreatment growth will affect lower incisor stability.

4. Overbite will increase posttreatment and will affect posttreatment incisor crowding.

5. The severity of posttreatment relapse is related to the degree of pretreatment crowding.

6. Changes in arch form are generally not stable postretention.

7. The lower incisors should be at 90° plus or minus 5° to the mandibular plane.

8 The effect of our treatment on the face overrides stability when deciding on premolar extractions.

If we are dealing with a growing child, a bonded mandibular retainer is placed (Fig. 5–1), and the patient is recalled annually.

After all growth is complete, and assuming we have been able to

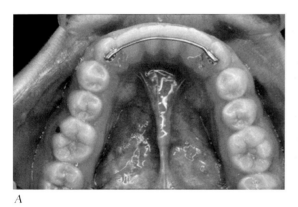
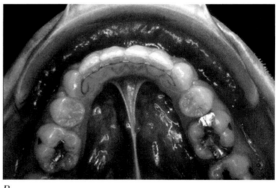

A   B

FIGURE 5–1   Two types of bonded retainers, an .036 bar and .0175 Respond wire.

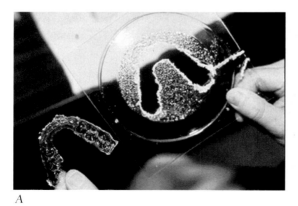
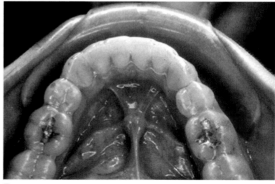

A   B

FIGURE 5–2   Removable retainers constructed of polypropylene using a Biostar machine.

meet all treatment objectives, the retainer is removed and an explanation of what happens to the lower incisors in nonorthodontic normal occulusions is presented. I use an analogy suggested by Parker:[29] "Teeth move as long as we live, just as surely as our hair color changes throughout our lives." If the patient is concerned about the occurrence of even the slightest change in alignment, then a set of removable retainers is constructed and the patient is instructed to wear them two or three nights a week indefinitely. A nominal charge is made for the retainers.

If we have compromised the stability of our treatment to provide the best in facial aesthetics, by changing arch form or moving lower incisors anteriorly, then a lifetime retention plan is prescribed at the posttreatment consultation. The patient is given the option of removable (Fig. 5–2) or fixed retainers and understands that all treatment hereafter will incur a charge. The majority of adult patients are encouraged to accept our lifetime retention plan.

Failure to charge for retention and retreatment encourages many orthodontists to let patients dismiss themselves from their practice after one or two years of retention, believing that "everything must be all right or they would have come back." Currently, approximately 30 percent of our patients are on a lifetime retention plan.

CONCLUSIONS

The extraction of premolars does not assure long-term stability of the lower incisors. Recent studies of postretention stability by different authors have produced significantly different results. It may be that the treatment goals and the mechanics used to reach those objectives differed in the populations studied. The studies by Little and others at the University of Washington are the most pessimistic. The study of Tweed technique cases by Sandusky is the most optimistic. Many other studies, notably those done at the University of Illinois by Sadowsky and others, fall somewhere in between. The methodology used at the University of Washington appears to be today's acceptable standard. Studies should be made of other populations using this approach.

As a clinical orthodontist with many years of experience, I am still striving for stability. To reduce the likelihood of relapse of the lower incisors, I have developed the following "Twelve Keys to Stability":

1. Whenever possible, allow the lower incisors to align themselves either through serial extraction or the use of a lip bumper in the early mixed dentition.

2. Overcorrect lower incisor rotations as early in treatment as possible.

3. Reproximation of incisors early in treatment and again at retention enhances stability (Fig. 5–3).

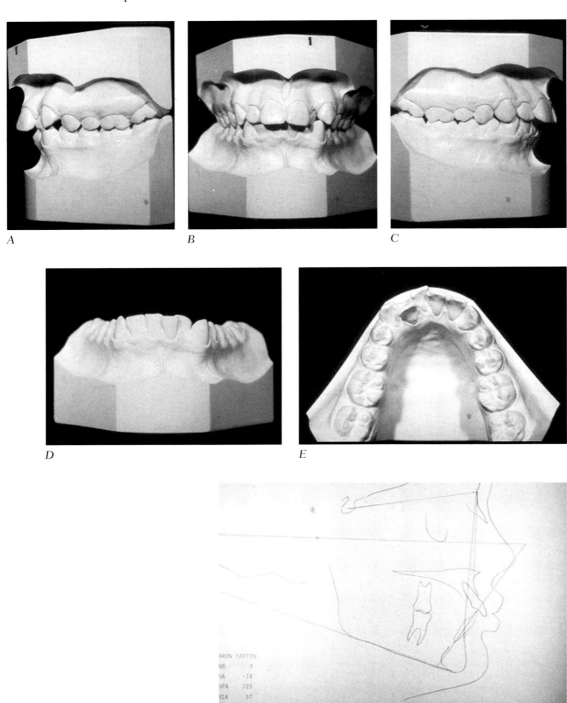

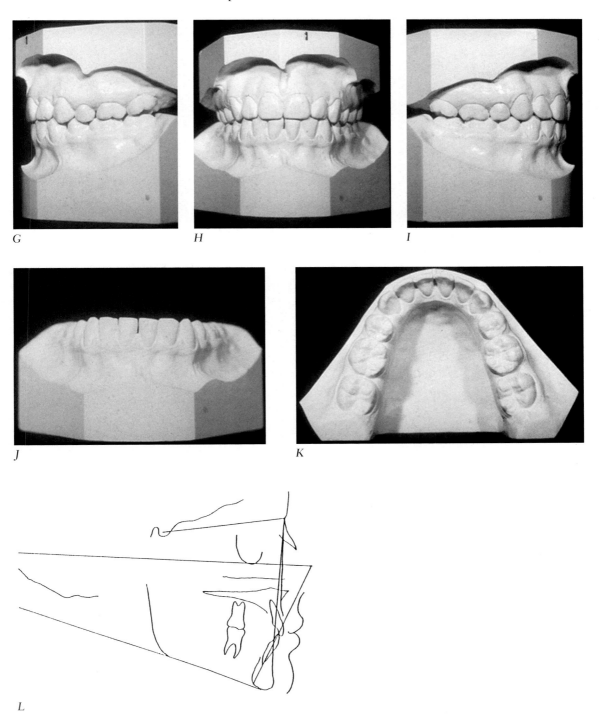

FIGURE 5–3   A case that meets all the requirements for stability.

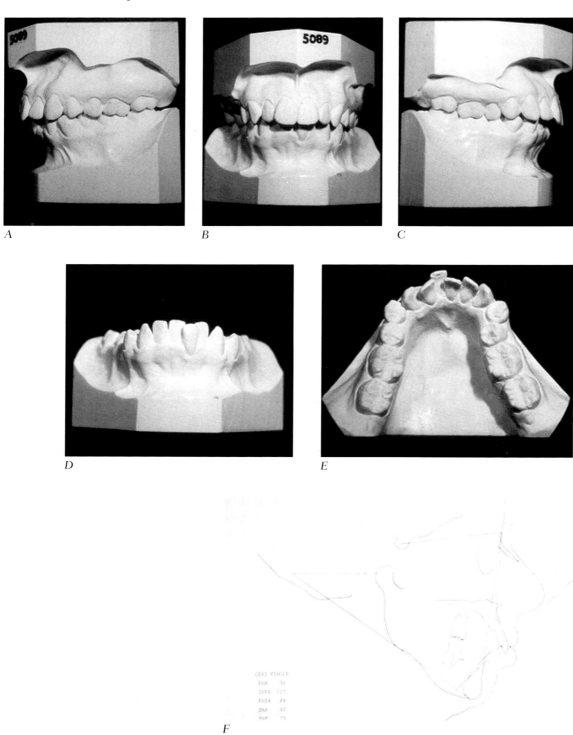

A

B

C

D

E

F

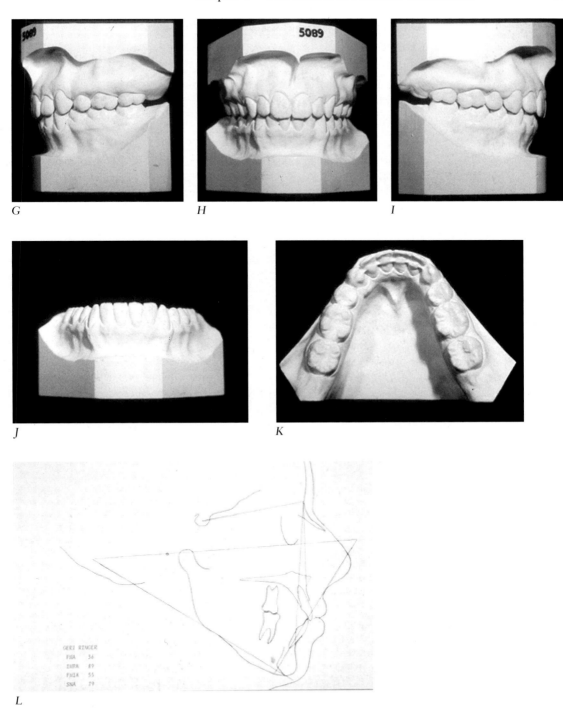

FIGURE 5–4   A case that will require lifetime retention.

4. Avoid increasing the intercanine width during active treatment.

5. Extract bicuspids in cases where mandibular arch discrepancy is 4 mm or greater, except where facial aesthetics dictates otherwise.

6. Recognize that the more a tooth is moved, the more likely it is to relapse, and overcorrect accordingly.

7. Upright lower incisors to at least 90° whenever the profile permits.

8. Create a flat occlusal plane during treatment, and overcorrect the overbite.

9. Prescribe supracrestal fiberotomy for severely rotated teeth.

10. Retain the lower arch until all growth is complete.

11. Place retainers the same day appliances are removed.

12. Recognize that compromise is often necessary in the interest of facial aesthetics and that sometimes lifetime retention (Fig. 5–4) is necessary.

Following these "Keys" will certainly not eliminate relapse: The only sure way is to prescribe lifetime retention for everyone. This seems impractical in light of the large number of patients seeking orthodontic treatment today.

I recently recalled a group of patients whose cases had been presented at meetings of the Tweed Foundation 10 or more years ago. At the time these cases were selected for presentation they were what I considered my best. I was pleased to find that the large majority of these patients had well-aligned lower incisors even though retention had been discontinued for many years.

REFERENCES

1. Proffit W: Contempory Orthodontics. St. Louis, C. V. Mosby, 1986, p.11.
2. Little R, Riedel R, Artun J: An evaluation of changes in mandibular anterior alignment from 10 to 20 years postretention. Am J Orthod Dentofacial Orthop 93:423–428, 1988.
3. Enlow D: Morphologic factors involved in the biology of relapse. J Charles H Tweed Foundation 8:16–23, 1980.
4. Angle E: Treatment of Malocclusion of the Teeth, 7th ed. Philadelphia, S. S White Dental Manufacturing Co, 1907.
5. Mershon J: Failures. Int J Orthod 22:338–342, 1936.
6. Hawley C: A removable retainer. Int J Orthod 2:291–298, 1919.
7. Begg P: Stone Age man's dentition. Am J Orthod 40:298–312, 1954.
8. Tweed C: Indications for the extraction of teeth in orthodontic procedure. Am J Orthod Oral Surg 30:405–428, 1944.
9. Tweed C: Clinical Orthodontics, Vol I. St. Louis, C. V. Mosby, 1966.
10. Tweed C: Interview with DS Brandt. J Pract Orthod 2:11–19, 1968.
11. Swanson W, Riedel R, D'Anna J: Postretention study: Incidence and stability of rotated teeth in humans. Angle Orthod 45:198–203, 1975.

12. Little R, Wallen T, Riedel R: Stability and relapse of mandibular anterior alignment—First premolar extraction cases treated by traditional edgewise orthodontics. Am J Orthod 80:349–65, 1981.
13. Shields T, Little R, Chapko M: Stability and relapse of mandibular anterior alignment: A cephalometric appraisal of first premolar extraction cases treated by traditional edgewise orthodontics. Am J Orthod 87:27–38, 1985.
14. Sinclair P, Little R: Maturation of untreated normal occlusions. Am J Orthod 83:114–123, 1983.
15. Little R: The Irregularity Index: A quantitative score of mandibular anterior alignment. Am J Orthod 68:554–563, 1975.
16. Little R, Riedel R: Postretention evaluation of stability and relapse-mandibular arches with generalized spacing. Am J Orthod 95:37–41, 1989.
17. Uhde M, Sadowsky C, Begole E: Long-term stability of dental relationships after orthodontic treatment. Angle Orthod 53:240–252, 1983.
18. Glenn G, Sinclair P, Alexander R: Nonextraction orthodontic therapy: Posttreatment dental and skeletal stability. Am J Orthod Dentofacial Orthop 92:321–328, 1987.
19. Gardner S, Chaconas S: Post-treatment and postretention changes following orthodontic therapy. Angle Orthod 46:151–161, 1976.
20. Sadowsky C, Sakois E: Long-term assessment of orthodontic relapse. Am J Orthod 82:456–463, 1982.
21. Sandusky WC: A long-term postretention study of Tweed extraction treatment. Master's thesis, University of Tennessee, 1983.
22. Davis T: A comparison of intercanine and intermolar width during treatment and three to five years postretention. Master's thesis, Ohio State University, 1971.
23. Kuftinic M, Strom D: Effects of edgewise treatment and retention on mandibular incisors. Am J Orthod 68:316–322, 1975.
24. El-Mangoury NH: Orthodontic relapse in subjects with varying degrees of anteroposterior and vertical dysplasia. Am J Orthod 75:548–581, 1975.
25. Sharpe W, Reed B, Subtelny J, Polson A: Orthodontic relapse, apical root resorption and crestal alveolar bone levels. Am J Orthod Dentofacial Orthop 91:252–258, 1987.
26. Reitan K: Principles of retention and avoidance of posttreatment relapse. Am J Orthod 55:776–90, 1969.
27. Edwards J: A surgical procedure to eliminate rotational relapse. Am J Orthod 57:35–46, 1970.
28. Boese L: Fiberotomy and reproximation without lower retention nine years in retrospect: Part 2. Angle Orthod 50:169–178, 1980.
29. Parker W: Retention—Retainers may be forever. Am J Orthod Dentofacial Orthop 95:505–513, 1989.

Stability and Relapse of Dental Arch Alignment

Robert M. Little

INTRODUCTION

For more than 35 years, the faculty and graduate students in the Department of Orthdodontics, University of Washington, have diligently collected diagnostic records of over 600 patients who a decade or more prior to that time had completed orthodontic treatment. Evaluation of satisfactory and unsatisfactory treatment has tested our theories, our personal biases, and our clinical convictions. Clinical practice is a balance of experience and our intuitive clinical experimentation, an evolving process that shapes our philosophy of treatment. Modifications of our methods and techniques can, and should, result from the range of treatment success as well as failures. In fact, we must be willing to examine our results critically, looking at those failures so that we can learn and improve. The key to successful practice of orthodontics is reexamining our treated patients and then carefully evaluating the results.

Of concern at the conclusion of treatment to both patient and practitioner is the degree of anticipated stability and the potential for relapse. When can retainer use be discontinued, and will significant change follow?

The focus of our research has been on the mandibular arch, the assumption being that alignment of the lower arch serves as a template around which the upper arch develops and functions. This chapter summarizes the results of this research on arch length problems and suggests clinical implications.

INADEQUATE ARCH LENGTH

EXTRACTION OF PREMOLARS IN THE FULL PERMANENT DENTITION

MATERIALS AND METHODS. Sixty-five sets of first premolar extraction patient records were evaluated pretreatment, posttreatment, and a minimum of 10 years postretention.[1,2] All cases had undergone a retention period, typically two years or more. A subsequent study was completed of 31 postretention cases a minimum of 20 years postretention.[3] In a later article, 32 second premolar extraction cases were evaluated.[4] Additionally, the role of third molars as a cause of postretention relapse was evaluated.[5]

RESULTS

1. Long-term alignment was highly variable and unpredictable (Fig. 6–1).
2. No characteristics, such as Angle classification, length of retention, patient age at the beginning of treatment, gender, or any measured variables such as initial or end of treatment alignment, overbite, overjet, arch width, or arch length, were of value in predicting the long-term result. No multiple correlations combining these variables improved our ability to predict the long-term stability or relapse of the cases.
3. Arch length and arch width typically decreased following retention as crowding increased. This seemed to occur in spite of treatment maintenance of the initial arch width, treatment expansion, or treatment constriction.
4. Success at maintaining satisfactory alignment was less than 30 percent, with nearly 20 percent demonstrating marked crowding many years after removal of retainers.
5. Pre- and posttreatment cephalometric data were of little value in predicting the long-term result. Combinations of cephalometric variables, such as incisor position and facial growth, were poor predictors of future arch irregularity. Postretention changes of cephalometric variables failed to explain crowding. Combinations of dental cast variables, descriptive characteristics, and cephalometric variables failed to show useful associations with long-term stability or relapse.
6. Arch length and arch width reduction with concomitant crowding continued well into the 20-to-30-years age span and apparently beyond, but the rate of change seemed to diminish after age 30.

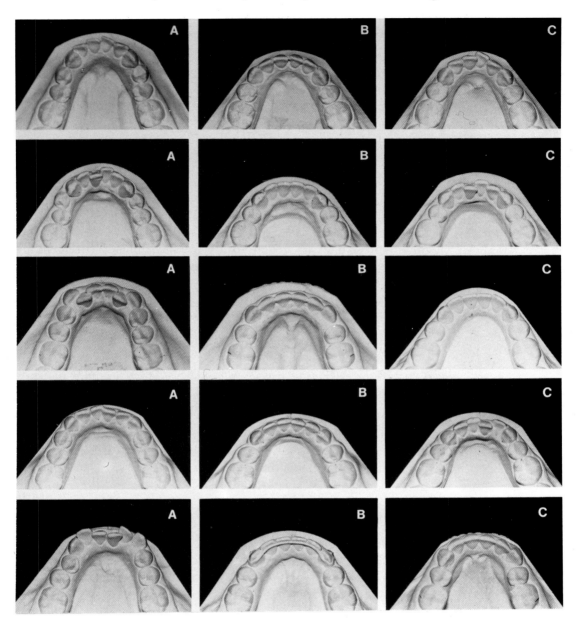

FIGURE 6–1   Results following premolar extraction, edgewise orthodontics, and retention. *A*, Pretreatment. *B*, End of active treatment. *C*, Postretention.

7. There appears to be no difference in treatment quality between first and second premolar extraction cases.

8. Third molar absence or presence, impacted or fully erupted, seemed to have little effect on the occurrence or degree of relapse.

SERIAL EXTRACTION OF DECIDUOUS TEETH PLUS PREMOLARS

MATERIALS AND METHODS. Thirty cases were evaluated following a series of mixed dentition extractions plus four first premolar extractions. All had undergone routine edgewise orthodontics, retention a minimum of two years, and had aged to qualify as a 10-year postretention case.[6] Fourteen cases of second premolar serial extraction were subsequently evaluated.[4]

RESULTS

1. Alignment usually improved during the physiologic drift stage following extraction of premolars and before the start of active treatment.
2. Serial extraction cases were no better aligned postretention than late extraction cases. Success was less than 30 percent.
3. Serial extraction cases were also unpredictable and highly variable relative to long-term alignment (Fig. 6–2).
4. As with late extraction cases, arch width and arch length typically decreased postretention.
5. There appears to be no difference in postretention quality between first and second premolar serial extraction cases.
6. No descriptive, cast, or cephalometric variables were useful predictors of long-term stability or relapse.

ARCH LENGTH INCREASE DURING THE MIXED DENTITION

MATERIALS AND METHODS. Twenty-six patients with records pretreatment, posttreatment, and a minimum of six years postretention were assessed. In all, arch length actively increased at least 1 mm during the mixed dentition with either fixed or removable appliances.[7]

RESULTS

1. Twenty out of 26 cases demonstrated a net loss of arch length compared to the initial measurement.

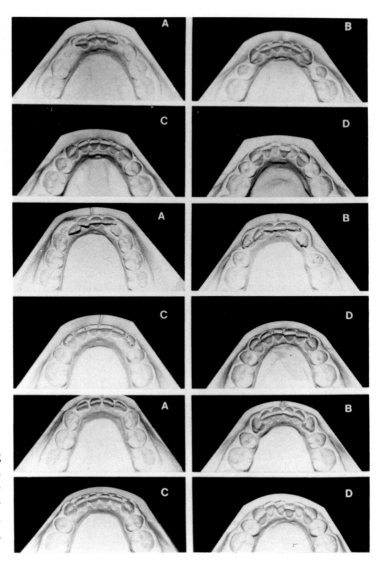

FIGURE 6–2   Results following first premolar serial extraction, physiologic drift, edgewise orthodontics, and retention. *A*, Preextraction. *B*, After physiologic drift. *C*, End of active treatment. *D*, Postretention.

2. Width constriction was a typical finding postretention.

3. Eighty-nine percent of cases demonstrated clinically unsatisfactory alignment at the postretention stage. Very few enlarged arches had acceptable long-term alignment. In fact, this sample showed a greater degree of relapse than all other samples examined from our files (Fig. 6–3).

4. Superimposition of cephalometric tracings showed variable direction and amount of molar and incisor change postretention. However, mesial molar movement, along with lingual tipping of incisors, were the most common cephalometric findings.

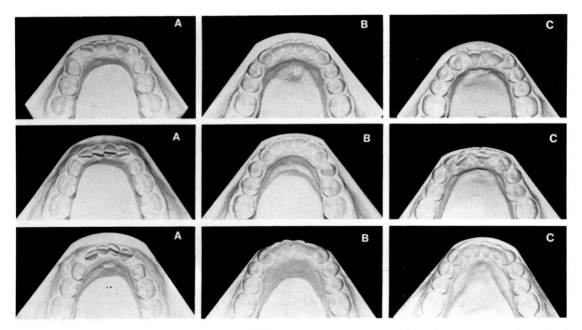

FIGURE 6–3   Results following nonextraction arch enlargement in the mixed dentition. *A*, Pretreatment. *B*, End of active treatment. *C*, Postretention.

ADEQUATE ARCH LENGTH

UNTREATED NORMAL OCCLUSIONS

MATERIALS AND METHODS. A sample of 65 "normal occlusion" cases all with serial records were evaluated utilizing the same criteria used with our treated cases. Dental casts and cephalometric radiographs were assessed for the mixed dentition and early permanent dentition and into early adulthood.[8,9]

RESULTS

1. As with treated cases, arch length and arch width typically decreased with time, a few cases progressing from "normal" to crowded by the early adult years.
2. Females showed the greater arch constriction trend and crowding tendency.
3. No single or multiple associations of clinical value were found when assessing stability or relapse versus cephalometric, dental cast, or descriptive variables.

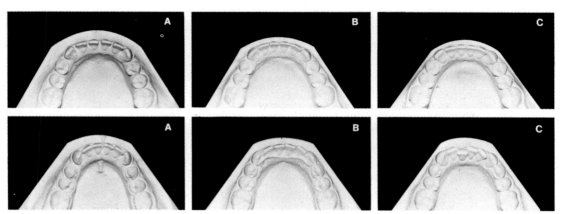

FIGURE 6–4 Generalized spacing cases treated nonextraction followed by retention. *A*, Pretreatment. *B*, End of active treatment. *C*, Postretention.

GENERALIZED SPACING

MATERIALS AND METHODS. Thirty cases with generalized spacing in the permanent dentition were evaluated pretreatment, posttreatment, and a minimum 10 years postretention. All had minimal or no rotated anterior teeth and minimal or no labiolingual deviations from "normal arch alignment" pretreatment. All had undergone edgewise orthodontics plus retention.[10]

RESULTS

1. Arch length decreased following treatment. In *every* case the final arch length was less than the initial value (Fig. 6–4).
2. Arch width decreases were noted in nearly all cases following treatment.
3. As a group, the sample had quite satisfactory postretention stability, with over half considered minimally irregular postretention.
4. Postretention overbite and overjet relapse averaged less than 1 mm, providing further evidence of the sample stability.
5. Spaces did not reopen in any case, further illustrating the constrictive trend of the sample.

CLINICAL IMPLICATIONS

It is apparent that arch width and arch length constriction with time is a normal physiologic process that routinely occurs following orthodontic treatment. The same process occurs with untreated patients as evidenced by our studies of untreated normal occlusions. This process continues well after the cessation of growth and can be quite active during the 20-to-30-years age span. From age 30 to 40 and beyond, the process seems to continue, but after age 30 the constrictive trend is much less. There is considerable patient variability, with a few individuals reaching a point of apparent stability by the late teenage years, but this is not typical. Most patients show active and significant changes for many years and even decades after the cessation of active treatment.

The degree of crowding that develops following retention is variable and unpredictable. Unfortunately, no factors, such as length of retention, age at the start of treatment, Angle classification, gender, or any dental cast or cephalometric measured variables, are useful predictors of future success or failure. Nor are any combinations of variables useful in improving predictability of the long-term result. Our patients and the parents of those young patients should be appraised beforehand of the liability for posttreatment change. They must understand clearly our limitations and their own role in the maintenance of the treated result. The orthodontist should not assume stability will occur but rather should assume that instability will likely be the pattern. Given such a posture, we can then plan against and prevent undesirable change.

PREMOLAR EXTRACTION. Removal of premolars to permit alignment of crowded teeth has been an accepted procedure for decades and continues as the most common treatment utilized for patients with crowded arches. In spite of achieving suggested and accepted cephalometric norms, and in spite of adhering to usual clinical standards of arch form, overbite, and so on, the long-term maintenance of acceptable results is disappointing, with only 30 percent of the patients demonstrating acceptable long-term results. Indefinite use of removable or fixed retainers, perhaps for life, seems to be the only logical recourse. Unfortunately, we do not yet know the undesirable sequella of such a retention program.

SERIAL EXTRACTION. Although crowding is usually reduced during the mixed and early permanent dentition following serial extraction, long-term evaluation shows results no better than with extraction after the premolars have fully erupted. Serial extraction still makes clinical sense to reduce the severity of the crowding pattern, to speed the follow-up orthodontic treatment, and to prevent erupting teeth from being blocked out of the band of attached gingiva. Long-term periodic retention or permanent retention seem to be the options that would ensure future success in maintaining the corrected result.

ARCH ENLARGEMENT OR "DEVELOPMENT." Anterioposterior and/or lateral increase in mandibular arch form usually fails, with the dental arch typically returning to the pretreatment size and shape. Most cases of mandibular arches "developed" during the mixed dentition fail, with postretention dimension less than pretreatment. Such a strategy requires permanent retention since success following retainer use is quite poor, with only 10 percent of patients with clinically acceptable results.

GENERALIZED SPACING. The most ideal long-term results were in this category, but unpredictable degrees of crowding occasionally occurred. Continuing observation of these patients beyond the typical retention stage is indicated, just as continuing recall and observation are warranted and prudent in all other types of treated malocclusions. As a group, the degree of relapse is much less in generalized spacing cases, but the practitioner does not know in advance which case will be the unusual one that demonstrates substantial relapse.

SUMMARY

Over time, decreasing mandibular dental arch dimensions in both treated and untreated malocclusions appears to be a normal physiologic phenomenon. The degree of arch length reduction, constriction, and resultant crowding is variable and unpredictable; however, several clinical guidelines are suggested:

1. Treat to ideal standards of perfection to obtain the best possible occlusion, oral health, and function.
2. Avoid enlargement of the lower arch unless mandated by facial profile concerns or to harmonize the occlusion with maxillary palatal expansion accomplished for cross-bite correction or unusual narrowness.
3. Use the patient's pretreatment arch form as a guide to arch shape.
4. Retain the arch form long term, and continue to monitor patient response into and throughout adult life.
5. Obtain the highest quality pre- and posttreatment records, and continue to utilize them to assess patient progress.

REFERENCES

1. Little R, Wallen T, Riedel R: Stability and relapse of mandibular anterior alignment—first premolar extraction cases treated by traditional edgewise orthodontics. Am J Orthod 80:349–365, 1981.
2. Shields T, Little R, Chapko M: Stability and relapse of mandibular anterior alignment—A cephalometric appraisal of first premolar extraction cases treated by traditional edgewise orthodontics. Am J Orthod 87:27–38, 1984.

3. Little R, Riedel R, Artun J: An evaluation of changes in mandibular anterior alignment from 10 to 20 years postretention. Am J Orthod Dentofacial Orthop 93:423–428, 1988.

4. McReynolds D, Little R: Mandibular second premolar extraction—Postretention evaluation of stability and relapse. Angle Orthod. 61:133–144, 1991.

5. Ades A, Joondeph D, Little R, Chapko M: A long-term study of the relationship of third molars to mandibular dental arch changes. Am J Orthod Dentofacial Orthop 97:323–325, 1990.

6. Little R, Riedel R, Engst, E: Serial extraction of first premolars—Postretention evaluation of stability and relapse. Angle Orthod 60:255–262, 1990.

7. Little R, Riedel R, Stein A: Mandibular arch length increase during the mixed dentition—Postretention evaluation of stability and relapse. Am J Orthod Dentofacial Orthop 97:393–404, 1990.

8. Sinclair P, Little R: Maturation of untreated normal occlusions. Am J Orthod 83:114–123, 1983.

9. Sinclair P, Little R: Dentofacial maturation of untreated normals. Am J Orthod 88:146–156, 1985.

10. Little R, Riedel R: Postretention evaluation of stability and relapse—Mandibular arches with generalized spacing. Am J Orthod Dentofacial Orthop 95:37–41, 1989.

Long-Term Stability Following Orthodontic Therapy

Cyril Sadowsky

INTRODUCTION

A lot of effort is made in the diagnosis and treatment planning of malocclusions, and rightly so. It is also usual to plan the retention objectives and to indicate the appropriate retention devices prior to commencing active treatment. However, the potential for relapse following orthodontic therapy is often considered in a somewhat abstract way, but should be of great concern to us as one of the important measures of the efficacy of our treatment.

In clinical practice, and even in teaching programs, clinical dogma exists regarding particular treatment strategies and specific intra-arch and interarch relationships that should be strived for in an effort to enhance stability in the retention and postretention stages. While these strategies are reasonable—for example, overcorrections, ideal inclinations and angulations, and maintenance of arch form—the expectations for long-term stability by excellent clinicians as opposed to those who have reviewed the subject or conducted independent research is somewhat different. The University of Connecticut symposium highlighted the anxiety existing within the profession when stability of orthodontic treatment is seriously questioned.

In the late 1970s, as part of a research contract sponsored by the National Institute of Dental Research, Bethesda, Maryland, on the long-term effects of orthodontic treatment, we at the Department of Orthodontics, College of Dentistry, University of Illinois at Chicago were able to gather longitudinal records of a sample of previously treated orthodontic patients who were recalled for a long-term follow-up evaluation. This chapter reviews some of the most important findings of that project, which considered stability of orthodontic treatment.

SAMPLE DESCRIPTION

From a pool of 1,800 previously treated cases, 158 patients responded to a recall letter, of whom 96 were examined and records taken. (The vast majority of the cases were from the offices of the late Dr. William B. Downs, Aurora, Illinois, and Dr. Abraham Goldstein, Chicago, Illinois; three faculty members also contributed cases.) All cases were treated to completion with full fixed appliances, usually followed by a Hawley retainer and a fixed lower lingual retainer for varying lengths of time. Fiberotomies were not performed, but some interproximal stripping may have been performed in a few cases. All patients had been treated 12 to 35 years previously with an average posttreatment time of 20 years. Prior to orthodontic treatment, 66 percent of cases exhibited Class II malocclusions and 34 percent Class I malocclusions; 61 percent were treated without extractions and 39 percent with extractions (Table 7–1).

FINDINGS

A malocclusion score was developed[1] to describe variations in interarch and intra-arch relationships, with an acceptable range of deviation from ideal being scored as zero. Overall analysis indicated that a marked improvement occurred from the pretreatment to long-term stages; however, the group as a whole reflected some long-term malocclusion (Table 7–2). Seventy-two percent of cases had a deviation that was outside the ideal range for at least one of the variables. Even though an excessive overjet (>3 mm) was present in 42 percent of cases at the long-term follow-up, it was the overbite that showed the least improvement over the long term as compared to pretreatment values. An excessive overbite (>3 mm) was present in 56 percent of cases pretreatment and in 41 percent of cases at the long-term stage (Table 7–3).

TABLE 7–1   Distribution of Original Malocclusion and Treatment Rendered

	Treatment Rendered		
Malocclusion	Extraction	Nonextraction	Total
Class I	14	19	33
Class II	23	40	63
Total	37	59	96

TABLE 7–2 Average Malocclusion Score at the Pretreatment and Long-Term Postretention Stages

	Pretreatment	*Long Term*
Mean	8.15	2.84
Standard deviation	3.20	2.74
Range	0–16	0–11

Pretreatment maxillary crowding was mild (0.5–3 mm) in 21 percent of cases, moderate (3.5–6 mm) in 10 percent of cases, and severe (6.5 mm or more) in 14 percent of cases; over the long term 38 percent had mild crowding, with no cases exhibiting moderate or severe crowding (Table 7–3).

Pretreatment mandibular crowding was mild in 26 percent, moderate in 20 percent, and severe in 16 percent of cases; long-term crowding was mild in 59 percent, moderate in 14 percent, and severe in 1 percent of cases (Table 7–3). When the lower incisor region was evaluated in greater detail using Little's Irregularity Index,[2] 33 percent of cases at the long-term stage were worse than at the pretreatment stage or had the same moderate (3.5–6 mm) or severe (>6 mm) irregularity as at pretreatment; 10 percent of cases improved from severe to moderate irregularity, 25 percent improved from severe or moderate pretreatment to mild long term (Table 7–4). When extraction and nonextraction cases were com-

TABLE 7–3 Malocclusion Scores and Frequencies at Pretreatment and Long-Term Postretention Stages (in percentages)

Variable	*Score*	*Pretreatment*	*Long Term*
Overjet (mm)			
0	0	0	3.2
0.5–3	0	22.9	54.2
3.5–6	2	43.8	40.6
6.5–9	3	17.7	1.0
9.5 or more	4	15.6	0
Not recorded		0	1.0
Overbite (mm)			
0	0	5.2	6.3
0.5–3	0	38.5	52.1
3.5–5	2	40.6	34.3
5.5 or more	3	15.6	6.3
Not recorded		0	1.0
Maxillary crowding (mm)			
0	0	55.2	62.5
0.5–3	0	20.8	37.5
3.5–6	2	10.4	0
6.5 or more	3	13.5	0
Mandibular crowding (mm)			
0	0	38.5	26.0
0.5–3	0	26.0	59.4
3.5–6	2	19.8	13.6
6.5 or more	3	15.6	1.0

TABLE 7–4   Distribution of Lower Incisor Irregularity at the Pretreatment and Long-Term Stages

| | Long Term | | | |
Pretreatment	Minimal	Moderate	Severe	Totals
Minimal	21	10	2	33 (50%)
Moderate	9	7	1	17 (25%)
Severe	8	7	2	17 (25%)
Totals	38 (57%)	24 (36%)	5 (7%)	67

TABLE 7–5   Lower Incisor Irregularity in Extraction and Nonextraction Cases at the Long-Term Stage

| | Irregularity Index (mm) | | |
Treatment Rendered	Mean	SD	t Value
Extraction (N = 24)	3.1	2.0	1.32 (ns)
Nonextraction (N = 53)	3.8	2.3	

ns: not significant ($p < 0.05$).

pared, there was no statistically significant difference in lower incisor irregularity at the long-term stage (Table 7–5).

Mean values for overjet, overbite, mandibular crowding, and mandibular intercuspid width at the pretreatment, posttreatment, and postretention stages are graphically shown for 45 nonextraction cases in Figure 7–1 and for 27 four-premolar-extraction cases in Figure 7–2). The trend for return to the pretreatment condition is readily apparent.[3]

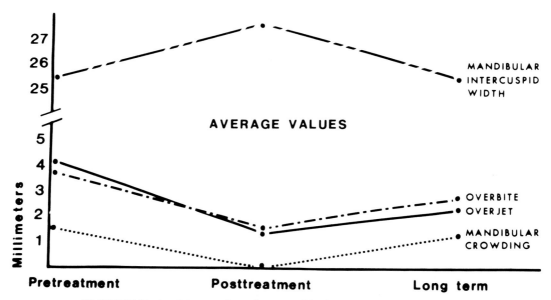

FIGURE 7–1   Mean values for mandibular intercuspid width, overbite, overjet, and mandibular crowding for 45 nonextraction cases before treatment and short and long term posttreatment. Standard deviations for all values were higher than the mean changes.

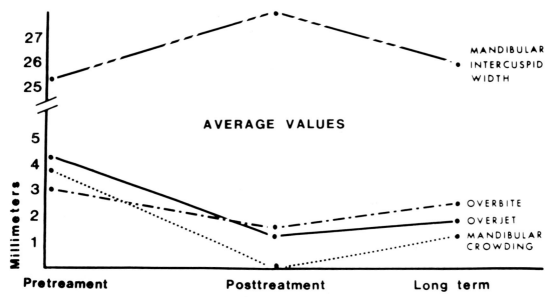

FIGURE 7–2   Mean values for mandibular intercuspid width, overbite, overjet, and mandibular crowding for 27 extraction cases before treatment and short and long term posttreatment. Standard deviations for all values were higher than the mean changes.

Using multiple-regression analysis, only 41 percent of the variability of lower incisor crowding over the long term could be accounted for by intra-arch and interarch changes posttreatment, with changes in the intercuspid width accounting for most (only 12 percent) of the variability.[3]

DISCUSSION

From the data presented in this report, including the more detailed previous publications referred to above and the publications of Little et al[4,5] from the University of Washington, Seattle, it is clear that when dental relationships of previously treated orthodontic patients are evaluated many years later, relapse occurs toward the pretreatment condition in a significant percentage of patients. Differences between the Illinois and Washington studies can be explained almost entirely on the basis of differences in the pretreatment malocclusions of the samples analyzed. Even though a moderately increased overjet, and more so an excessive overbite, appears to be present in many cases, the most noticeable deviations from ideal involve lower incisor irregularity. When the results from the various studies are compared in detail, it is interesting how similar the findings are. These differences are to a large degree also reflected in the fact that the Illinois sample is predominantly nonextraction treatment with a predominance of Class II malocclusions, whereas the Washington sample reported to date represents only extraction therapy. Furthermore, in a recent study[6] of a sample of 42 cases that were followed up many years later, in which all first premolars had been extracted as the sole treatment of space deficiency in the middle or early permanent dentition, the degree of malocclusion was almost identical to that reported in our study.[1] Even in a sample of 35 children who received treatment only in the maxillary arch in which first premolars were extracted,[7] a mean of 2.5 mm (standard deviation 1.52) crowding of the lower anterior teeth was observed four years postretention; this crowding was greater than that observed in a group of 19 untreated children over a similar period.

While findings of this nature may appear disturbing to clinicians, we should be consoled by the fact that orthodontic treatment produces a marked improvement in dental relationships with significant aesthetic benefits in the overwhelming majority of patients. Some change posttreatment is acceptable and of no real concern. It is equally apparent that our expectations and those of our patients should be reasonable and clearly understood prior to initiation of treatment and reinforced during the retention phase. Explanations for this relapse are many and varied, and our ability to reliably predict the long-term outcome is not good. Even though the findings generally indicate a decrease in the intercanine width posttreatment, this change accounts for only 12 percent of the variability in lower incisor crowding; when all study model variables are considered, only 41 percent of the variability in lower incisor crowding can be accounted for.

These seemingly pessimistic findings must not engender a negative attitude and are not a license to provide inferior treatment by "straightening the front teeth, letting the patient chew gum, and letting the chips fall where they will." To the contrary, once the decision has been made to provide comprehensive orthodontic treatment, it is our obligation to provide the best possible treatment for the patient in an attempt to achieve as ideal a result as possible, paying attention to details, including overcorrections. Even though the study of four-premolar extraction cases by Persson et al[6] reported similar overall findings to the Illinois study, many interarch and intra-arch relationships were not compared; furthermore, the nature of the pretreatment malocclusions was different. It is to be hoped that the inclusion of a well-thought-out retention plan will enhance our ability to improve long-term stability. One of the few reported studies of good long-term stability was that by Boese,[8] in which marked stability of the lower anterior segment was shown four to nine years posttreatment in 40 cases treated with the extraction of four premolars; all cases had circumferential supracrestal fiberotomies and reproximation without retention. Fiberotomies and reproximation should be resorted to in many cases in the hope of enhancing long-term stability.

With this type of information available, it appears that it would be prudent to consider many years of fixed retention in many patients, with some needing permanent retention. The need for a removable retainer that is worn occasionally and indefinitely should also be considered in some cases. Patients must be informed of the potential for relapse and be given some of the responsibility for monitoring long-term stability.

Acknowledgment: I would like to dedicate this chapter to the memory of the late Dr. William B. Downs and to Dr. Abraham Goldstein for their dedication to orthodontics and their efforts in accumulating records, without which this project would not have been possible.

REFERENCES

1. Sadowsky C, Sakols EI: Long-term assessment of orthodontic relapse. Am J Orthod 82:456–463, 1982.
2. Puneky PJ, Sadowsky C, Begole EA: Tooth morphology and lower incisor alignment many years after orthodontic therapy. Am J Orthod 86:299–305, 1984.
3. Uhde MD, Sadowsky C, Begole EA: Long-term stability of dental relationships after orthodontic treatment. Angle Orthod 53:240–252, 1983.
4. Little RM, Wallen TR, Riedel RA: Stability and relapse of mandibular anterior alignment—First premolar extraction cases treated by traditional edgewise orthodontics. Am J Orthod 80:349–365, 1981.
5. Little RM, Riedel RA, Artun, J: An evaluation of changes in mandibular anterior alignment from 10 to 20 years postretention. Am J Orthod Dentofacial Orthop 93:423–428, 1988.
6. Persson M, Persson E, Skagius S: Long-term spontaneous changes following removal of all first premolars in Class I cases with crowding. Eur J Orthod 11:271–282, 1989.
7. Owman G, Bjerklin K, Kurol J: Mandibular incisor stability after orthodontic treatment in the upper arch. Eur J Orthod 11:341–350, 1989.
8. Boese LR: Fiberotomy and reproximation without lower retention—Nine years in retrospect. Part II. Angle Orthod 50:169–178, 1980.

Treatment and Retention for Long-Term Stability

Richard G. "Wick" Alexander

This chapter is based on my 30 years of clinical experience in treating over 10,000 patients with fixed appliances. Some of my statements are documented in the literature, but other observations have come from following many patients and comparing those who have remained stable with those who have relapsed.

RETENTION BEGINS WITH DIAGNOSIS AND TREATMENT PLANNING!

GOALS IN DIAGNOSIS AND TREATMENT PLANNING

Treatment goals include:

1. Balanced soft tissue profile.
2. Nonextraction treatment when possible.
3. Mandibular incisors upright on basal bone.
4. Good interincisal angle.
5. Normal root artistic positioning.
6. Mandibular molars upright.
7. Cuspids not expanded.

8. Normal overbite and overjet.

9. Class I cuspids—cuspid protected occlusion.

Although the majority of cases are now treated nonextraction, the final decision depends upon five major factors:

1. Soft tissue profile.

2. Arch length discrepancy.

3. Position of the mandibular incisors.

4. Growth potential.

5. Periodontal condition.

CEPHALOMETRIC GUIDES

Cephalometric measurements are important guides, but should not be taken as "final truths." Emphasis is placed upon the vertical and sagittal growth dimensions. These dimensions are identified to determine the amount and direction of the patient's skeletal growth.

The mandibular incisor position is observed, and a decision made as to where its final position should be. Let's talk about IMPA. Where is the most stable position? Is it 90°–95°, à 1a Tweed? Tweed stated that "the lower incisors should be upright on the basal bone."

It has been my observation that "stable" is the position in which the patient presents. A stable range for mandibular incisors can be from 70° to 110°.

The mandibular incisors can be uprighted a great amount (Tweed) and remain stable. In his unpublished thesis at Baylor University, Dr. Sam Papandreas studied the amount of drift that takes place when four first bicuspids are extracted in Class I malocclusions and treatment is initiated only on the maxillary arch. This "driftodontics" of the mandibular teeth demonstrated some interesting results.

Dr. Papandreas found that on an annualized basis:

1. The mandibular anteriors uprighted an average of 8°.

2. The cuspids drifted distally and expanded 1.7 mm.

3. The molars drifted forward only 1.2 mm.

Also at Baylor, Dr. Chris Nevant's thesis on lip bumpers showed some interesting results regarding the advancement of mandibular incisors. In 40 patients (20 each from two practices), the mandibular incisors tipped labially 1.4 mm, 3° in each case. Does this indicate that an anterior limit exists as to how far the incisors can be advanced and still be in the stable position?

INTERINCISAL ANGLE

In addition to torque control of the mandibular incisors, the maxillary incisors and their relationship to the mandibular incisors must be addressed. To maintain the corrected overbite, good maxillary torque and interincisal angle must be established during treatment.

MANDIBULAR FIRST MOLAR POSITION

In deep-bite cases, the permanent correction of overbite is also related to the ability to upright, or tip back, the mandibular first molars. By uprighting the first molars, several good things happen: (1) Anterior arch length is gained; (2) second premolars are simultaneously extruded to help level the mandibular arch; and (3) posterior occlusal stops are established to prevent anterior overbite relapse.

ANGULATION (ARTISTIC POSITIONING) OF MANDIBULAR INCISORS

Raleigh Williams observed that the mandibular laterals should be positioned with more angulation in order to improve stability.

Clinical observation of posttreatment patients over the years has led me to agree that one of the causes of relapse in the mandibular anterior arch has been the poor artistic positioning of the mandibular lateral incisors. If the incisal edges of the mandibular anteriors are aligned evenly, the laterals will be too upright. If, however, the lateral roots are aligned more parallel to the cuspid root, then relapse seems to be less severe.

MUSCULATURE

Oral musculature has an obvious effect upon stability and relapse. A normal skeletal pattern with no abnormal muscular habits can help make the end result and the orthodontist look very good. When the growth and muscular patterns are divergent, however, the orthodontist's limitations become glaringly obvious. Muscular factors that affect tooth stability include:

1. Tight lip musculature.
2. Placid lip musculature.
3. Tongue thrusting.
4. Mouth breathing.
5. Thumb sucking.

The vertical skeletal pattern with tongue thrusting and mouth breathing habits seems to be the most difficult problem to correct and maintain. Relapse is not uncommon in these patients.

ACTIVE TREATMENT

After carefully evaluating a patient's malocclusion and skeletal pattern, including factors already mentioned, and setting goals for the treatment objectives, orthodontic treatment is initiated. The philosophy of treatment should be, "Begin with the end in mind."

Although all of the goals mentioned can be achieved with basically any edgewise orthodontic appliance, it makes sense to incorporate as many of these factors as possible into the design of a "straight-wire" appliance. After proper diagnosis and treatment planning have taken place, an appliance has been designed that will place the teeth in positions to help eliminate relapse. Appliance design and placement can have a lasting effect upon the position of the teeth.

In this treatment technique, a step-by-step sequence is designed to get the patient into finishing archwires as rapidly as possible. Once properly positioned, the teeth are held for a long period of time before appliances are removed. This facilitates stability. The appliance has an 0.018 slot, and the finishing archwire is routinely 0.017 × 0.025 stainless steel.

APPLIANCE DESIGN FEATURES FOR STABILITY

- Anterior bracket torque to achieve proper interincisal angle
  a. Maxillary incisors
     1. Centrals   14°
     2. Laterals   7°
  b. Mandibular incisors
     1. Centrals   −5 °
     2. Laterals   −5°
- Bracket angulation to achieve stable mandibular anteriors
  a. Mandibular incisors
     1. Centrals   2°
     2. Laterals   6°
- Bracket angulation to achieve good posterior stops
  b. Mandibular first molars   −6°
- Bracket angulation to prevent relapse at extraction sites
  c. Extraction of first bicuspids   −3° on second bicuspids
  d. Extraction of second bicuspids   −3° on first bicuspids

• Bracket height to achieve stable overbite
  Measured parallel to the bracket slot from the incisal or occlusal edge.
  a. Normal/deep bite

OPEN BITE

Open bite problems deserve special attention. The first problem to address is the abnormal tongue position.

MYOFUNCTIONAL THERAPY. As an alternative to myofunctional therapy, the following program is taught to anterior tongue-thrust patients:

First, the patient must learn to "click." This procedure involves the patient's putting the tip of the tongue on the roof of the mouth and snapping it off the palate to produce a clicking sound. The tongue position on the palate during this activity approximates the tongue position when swallowing properly. In addition, the patient must practice making a slurred sound, in which he or she sucks air into the roof of the mouth around the tongue. During this exercise, the tongue naturally positions itself into the anterior palatal vault. The patient then presses the tip of the tongue at this position and swallows, while squeezing the teeth together.

After active treatment, an additional swallowing aid is provided for the patient. A hole approximately 3–4 mm in diameter is placed in the maxillary retainer at the point where the tip of the tongue should be placed during swallowing.

Open bite problems are treated in an opposite manner from deep-bite cases. Rather than upright mandibular molars, in open bite cases, the molars are tipped forward. Rather than level the mandibular arch, an accentuated curve of Spee is placed in the archwire.

The anterior teeth are extruded rather than intruded, and the posterior teeth are intruded rather than extruded. These goals are accomplished by:

1. 0° or +6°-tip for mandibular first molars.

2. Increasing bracket height by 0.5–1 mm on anterior teeth out of occlusion.

3. Decreasing bracket height by 0.5–1 mm on posterior teeth in occlusion.

4. Placing opposite curves of Spee in archwires.

5. Using vertical anterior elastics.

Most tongue-thrust patients wear anterior box elastics at some time during treatment. Patients are told that every time the tongue touches the elastics, they are tongue thrusting. This signals them to concentrate on the proper swallowing pattern by moving the tongue away from the elastics and into the anterior palatal vault.

OVERCORRECTION OF ROTATIONS

When using a single bracket with wings on a tooth that is severely rotated, the wing in the direction of the rotation can be removed. The bracket can then be positioned properly, with the remaining wing serving to rotate the tooth into proper position. The removed wing is never replaced. Often the tooth will overrotate, but this is good because overrotation guards against post-treatment relapse.

CIRCUMFERENTIAL SUPRACRESTAL FIBEROTOMY

Rotated teeth, when corrected, seem to have a memory: They have a tendency to return to their original positions. The transseptal fibers are often the specific cause of dental relapse. These fibers are stretched during treatment. After appliances are removed, the fibers tend to contract, returning the periodontal membrane and hence the dentition toward its original configuration.

In adolescent patients with typically crowded pretreatment conditions, if these teeth are held in place with retainers after treatment, the fibers seem to reshape to conform to the new dental configuration. Therefore, posttreatment and postretention relapse are minimized. An exception to this pattern is when maxillary laterals are positioned lingually prior to treatment, a significant tendency for relapse remains. Other exceptions include severely rotated teeth and previously impacted teeth.

Adult patients cannot expect significant reconfiguration of the transseptal fibers during active treatment and retention. Therefore, in adult patients the circumferential supracrestal fiberotomy is a routine procedure. This surgery is performed six weeks prior to bond removal. As a result, the transseptal fiber memory is reduced, preventing significant relapse.

COUNTDOWN TO RETENTION

All of the procedures just described are performed during treatment to place the teeth in positions that will maintain the most stable results. Now it is time for the "countdown to retention."

The countdown is initiated when active orthodontic treatment is complete. Ten criteria must be met in order for a patient to be deemed ready for retention:

1. Coincidence of centric relation and centric occlusion.
2. Class I cuspid relationship.
3. Maintenance of mandibular cuspid width.
4. Interincisal angle close to the norm, with proper torque in both maxillary and mandibular incisors.
5. Normal anterior overbite and overjet.
6. Normal buccal overjet.
7. Leveled maxillary and mandibular arches.
8. All spaces closed; all rotations eliminated.
9. Roots parallel near extraction sites.
10. Posterior cusps may or may not be settled.

This phase of treatment lasts six weeks, during which final detailing and settling can be accomplished. Posterior settling is done using one of three approaches: (1) sectioning the mandibular arch only; (2) sectioning the maxillary arch only; or (3) sectioning both arches.

To section the mandibular arch, cut the archwire distal to the cuspids on both sides and remove the posterior sections. For cuspid settling, section the maxillary arch distal to the laterals. Otherwise, section distal to the cuspids.

For Class II deep bite cases, section the mandibular arch only, and initiate the use of 3/4-inch, 2-ounce elastics in a "W with a tail" configuration. The posterior bite is stabilized so that the anterior overbite will be less likely to relapse. The elastics are worn 24 hours a day for three weeks. In addition to wearing the elastics, patients are asked to chew sugarless gum to further settle the bite.

For Class III and open bite cases, the maxillary arch is sectioned. The 3/4-inch, 2-ounce elastics are worn in an "M with a tail" configuration. Additional overbite correction can be achieved by utilizing anterior up-and-down elastics. For Class I cases, the elastics are worn without a "tail."

In summary, the countdown to retention finalizes the occlusion before the appliances are removed. Depending upon the need, the wires are sectioned and elastics placed, giving a Class II vector (W with a tail), a Class III vector (M with a tail), a Class I up-and-down vertical vector (M or W without a tail), or a combination of any of these. Anterior box elastics are used when additional overbite is required. Final cusp interdigitation and anterior overbite are achieved.

BAND REMOVAL AND RETENTION

The next step is the band removal appointment. After all of the bands and brackets are removed, impressions are taken on the maxillary and mandibular arches.

Active retention normally utilizes a maxillary wraparound retainer and a mandibular 3 × 3, either banded or bonded. The retainers are designed to eliminate occlusal interferences and to allow for continuing vertical settling.

The day after the band removal appointment, the patient returns for the retainers to be seated. The retainers are worn 24 hours a day.

The patient's next appointment is scheduled six weeks after the bands and brackets are removed. The retainer is adjusted, and the teeth are artistically recontoured. The patient continues to wear the retainer 24 hours a day.

Three months postremoval, the patient's final records are taken, which include photos and a cephalometric X-ray.

The third retainer adjustment appointment takes place approximately 4.5 months postremoval. The patient is instructed to wear the retainer at night only. The next appointment is scheduled for 12 months later.

One year later, the retainer is adjusted, and the patient is instructed to continue wearing it at night only. By this time, the third molars are discussed. The wisdom teeth should be resolved as quickly as possible. If the X-rays indicate the need for extraction, they should be removed as soon as the oral surgeon sees fit.

Annual observation continues until after the third molars have been removed. The mandibular 3 × 3 retainer normally remains in place a minimum of three years. At the time the mandibular 3 × 3 is removed, interproximal enamel reduction is performed from cuspid to cuspid. The final appointment is scheduled one year after the 3 × 3 removal to observe any possible relapse.

INVISIBLE RETAINER

An alternative to the maxillary wraparound retainer and 3 × 3 are removable, full-coverage clear acrylic appliance. This design can also be used as a "one-tooth" positioner in selected cases.

LIFETIME RETENTION

For years, my philosophy has been to never tell the patient to stop wearing the retainer. Releasing the patient forever is a difficult and often emotional experience. Patient should never be told, "This is it. Don't come back. It's all over." I tell him or her,

Officially, we're releasing you as a patient. But I want you to do one more thing for me. Every Sunday night, just for old times' sake, I want you to wear your upper retainer. If you do that, those teeth are going to stay beautiful for the rest of your life. Now, if you don't wear that retainer, there is a possibility those teeth can shift. It's a decision you have to make. You're going to be your own orthodontist from here on out. It's up to you.

If you ever break a retainer, you can always call us and we will be glad to make you a new one. But there is no way we can guarantee your teeth will stay beautifully straight unless you keep wearing the retainer from time to time.

Few patients actually wear the retainer after they are released, but I like to let them know that I want them to wear it. My final sentence is, "If you ever have any problems with your teeth, be sure to come back to see us."

As long as the patient's dentist feels that no periodontal problems occur, I have no problems with a patient with good oral hygiene habits continuing to wear his bonded 3 × 3 indefinitely.

RELAPSE

Approximately 80 percent of my cases experience no significant relapse. Another 15 percent relapse only very slightly, and about 5 percent show meaningful relapse.

POSSIBLE SOURCES OF RELAPSE

Many variables exist over which the orthodontist has no control. Poor skeletal patterns and abnormal muscular, sleeping, and other habits can have a great influence upon the long-term stability of the finished case.

Possibly the most common cause of orthodontic relapse, however, is poor treatment. Improper diagnosis and treatment and/or less than desired results can have no other fate.

Dr. Jim McNamara stated that "the more functionally stable the result, the less posttreatment changes occur." These are words of wisdom.

An additional source of relapse is the mishandling of the third molars. Although it is not certain whether third molar eruption is ever responsible for mandibular anterior relapse, the potential impact cannot be ignored. Therefore, orthodontic treatment is not complete until the third molar issue has been resolved.

As discussed earlier, another source of relapse is periodontal memory, or the tendency of teeth to return to their original positions. To reduce this tendency, I routinely recommend that a circumferential supracrestal fiberotomy (CSF) be performed six weeks before the appliances are removed. A CSF is recommended in adolescent patients when the maxillary laterals are positioned lingually or if severe rotations were present before treatment. In adult patients, the CSF is a routine procedure.

POSTTREATMENT STABILITY

A study by Dr. Gayle Glenn, published in the *American Journal of Orthodontics* in October 1987, revealed some interesting findings. She analyzed 28 nonextraction cases randomly selected from my practice. Of the 28 cases, 14 were Class I and 14 were Class II, Division 1. The average pretreatment age was 12 years, 7 months. The average posttreatment age was 14 years, 9 months. And the average postretention age at the time of the study was 26 years, 7 months. Therefore, active treatment time was 2 years, 2 months; active retention time was 3 years, 11 months; and the mean postretention time was 7 years, 11 months.
The results of this study concluded:

MANDIBULAR CUSPID EXPANSION. Cuspids were expanded by an average of 0.6 mm in the sample during treatment. The average cuspid width decreased 1 mm posttreatment.

MANDIBULAR MOLAR EXPANSION. The study revealed that intermolar width had been increased 1.1 mm, and this expansion was maintained posttreatment. Clinically, this can be called buccal uprighting.

REDUCING OVERJET AND OVERBITE. Long-term reduction of overjet in these cases was 3.3 mm. The original overbite averaged 4.6 mm and was corrected to 2.7 mm. No significant change took place postretention.

INTERINCISAL ANGLE. The interincisal angle averaged 129.7° pretreatment. After treatment, it had changed to 132°. Postretention found no significant changes.

MANDIBULAR INCISOR POSITION. In Dr. Glenn's study, IMPA averaged 94.5° in pretreatment. In these nonextraction cases, IMPA was 94.8° after treatment. Postretention eight years later showed IMPA at 95.1°.

IRREGULARITY INDEX. Pretreatment mandibular incisor irregularity in this study ranged from 1 to 6 mm. Twenty-four cases exhibited minimal incisor irregularity at postretention. Three had moderate relapse, and one has severe relapse. Why this case failed so badly is unknown. To be sure, though, it is that one case that keeps the orthodontist humble.

SHAPE AND STABILITY OF MANDIBULAR ARCH FORM

A study by Dr. Mark Felton concerning stability of arch form was published in the *American Journal of Orthodontics* in December 1987. His sample included mandibular dental casts on 90 cases. These cases were divided in the following manner: (1) 30 skeletal and dental Class I nonextraction orthodontically treated cases; (2) 30 skeletal and dental Class II nonextraction orthodontically treated cases; and (3) 30 untreated normal cases (taken from Dr. Larry Andrews' sample).

Arch forms were generated for each sample and compared to 17 commercially produced arch forms.

A shape representing a combination of the "Par" and "Vari-Simplex" arch forms approximated 50 percent of the cases in the three samples. The remaining 50 percent displayed a wide variety of arch forms. Changes in arch form during treatment were not always stable; almost 70 percent showed long-term posttreatment changes.

Although we continue to seek the ideal arch form, the results of this study supported the concept that there is no single, universal ideal arch form applicable to all cases.

Dr. Felton concluded that no one arch form can be expected to fit every dental arch. Individual customizing is necessary in many cases to obtain stable orthodontic results.

CHANGING TREATMENT PHILOSOPHIES MAY ALTER CONCEPTS OF RETENTION

Historically, U.S. orthodontic education has taught to not expand the arches transversely. Increase of intercanine and intermolar width does not remain stable. A different approach to treatment, however, may dispel that truism.

In the past six years, I have been exploring with outstanding success the transverse dimension by the use of rapid palatal expanders and lip bumpers in severely crowded arches. This treatment modality allows the case to be treated with a full complement of teeth (nonextraction) without adversely affecting the soft tissue profile.

The unanswered question in cases in which this treatment approach is used is that of long-term stability. The answer lies in the future.

CONCLUSION

When the retainers are removed, if the teeth have been placed in the appropriate positions during active treatment, interproximal reduction is properly performed, and wisdom teeth are resolved, the chances of the result remaining stable are excellent.

Retention is as important as active treatment in producing an outstanding and lasting quality orthodontic result. It is usually a three-year process, during which the clinician should remain in control of the case and encourage the patient to continue wearing the retainers. The only way that retention can be successful is for the patient to have been treated first to a normally balanced occlusion. To expect little or no posttreatment relapse, the orthodontic result must include:

1. Teeth kept within the alveolar trough.
2. The mandibular arch leveled.
3. Proper interincisal angle.
4. Balanced occlusal stops.
5. Wisdom teeth resolved.

A comprehensive retention program can make all the difference in the world to the final result the patient can receive.

CASE REPORT

The following case report spans 21 years.

Patient S. T. was a 10-year, 7-month-old female who presented with a Class II skeletal pattern, a mandibular arch length discrepancy of 6 mm, an overbite of 5 mm, and an overjet of 10 mm.

She was treated nonextraction with cervical headgear and full banded appliances. She was a cooperative patient. Her poor growth pattern resulted in acceptable results (for that time in my career) (Figs. 8–1 and 8–2).

Fifteen years later, S. T. returned to the office requesting a new maxillary retainer because of a slightly rotated maxillary right lateral incisor (Fig. 8–3).

In studying this patient's long-term results, two interesting findings were observed. The bad news was the relapsed (or possibily never corrected) Class II skeletal pattern. The good news, however, was that the mandibular arch, although crowded in pretreatment (6 mm), was surprisingly stable, and the mandibular incisors advanced in treatment by 4° (IMPA). The cause of this, in the author's opinion, was the patient's continuing to wear her maxillary retainer once or twice a month throughout posttreatment.

During reexamination, possible future treatment, including orthognathic surgery, was discussed with the patient. The treatment plan was accepted.

FIGURE 8–1

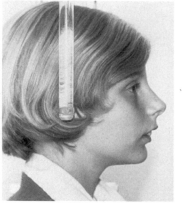
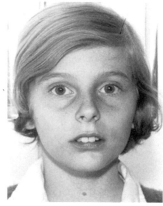

Patient: S.T. No. 1332

Age: 10 yrs. 7 mos.

Profile: Class II

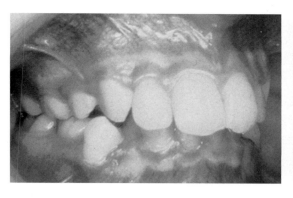
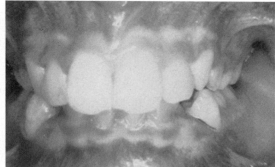

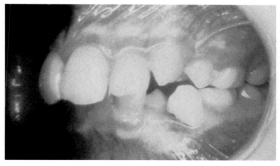
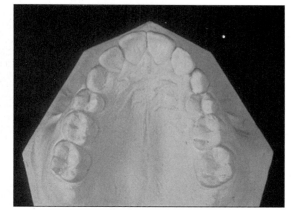

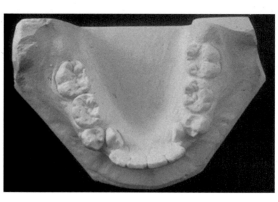

(Continued)

FIGURE 8–1   *(Continued)*

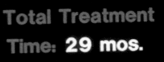

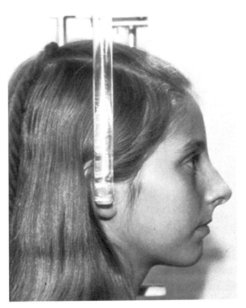

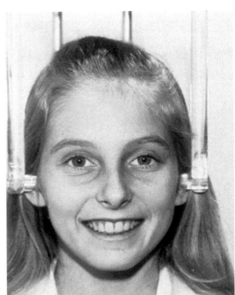

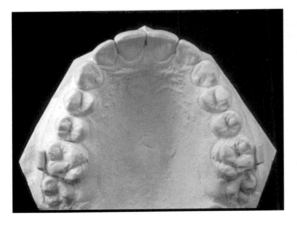

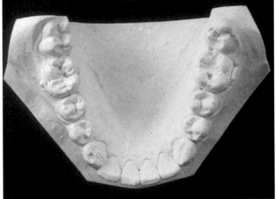

FIGURE 8–1 *(Continued)*

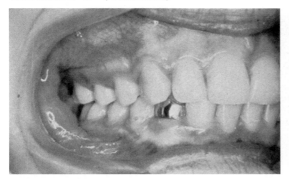
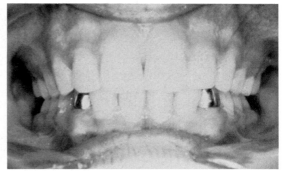
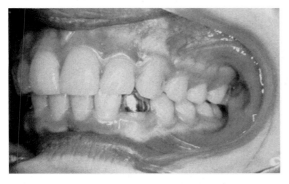

FIGURE 8–2

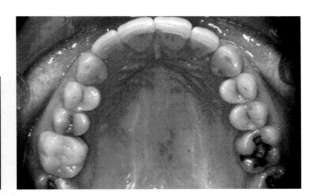

15 YEARS
POST - TREATMENT

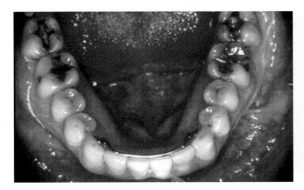
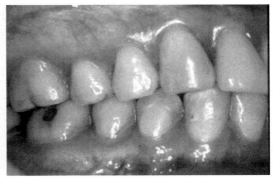

(Continued)

FIGURE 8–2   *(Continued)*

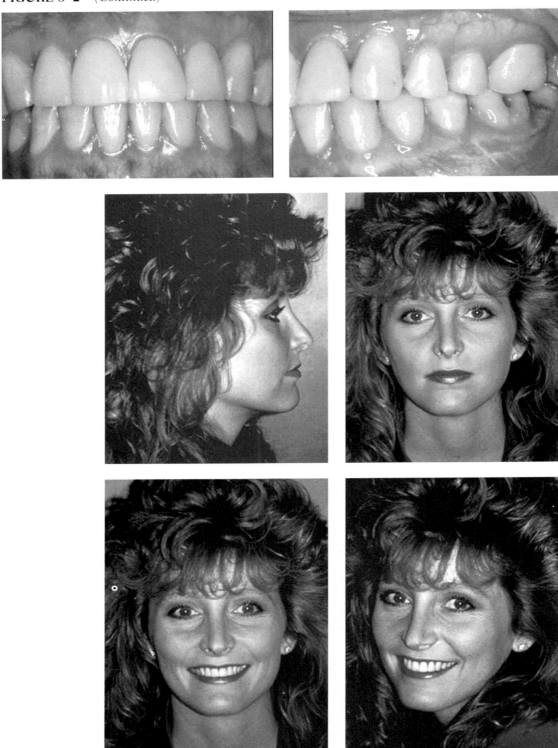

FIGURE 8–3

2 YEARS POST – TREATMENT (RETREATMENT)

Chief Concern: "Large Nose and Deficient Chin"

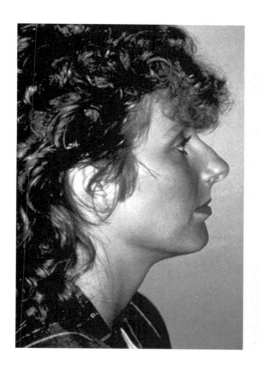
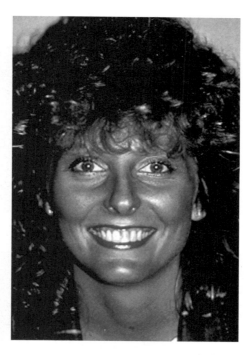

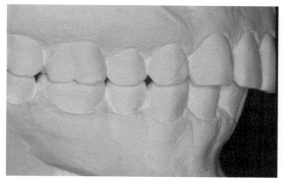
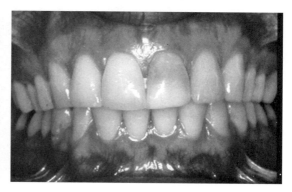

(*Continued*)

FIGURE 8–3   (*Continued*)

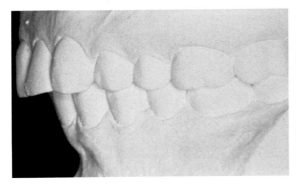
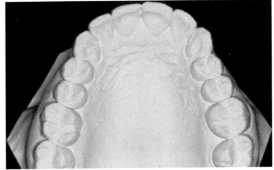
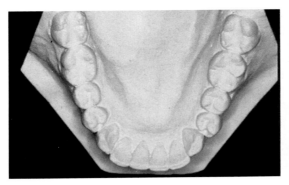
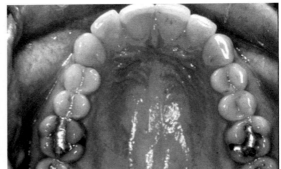
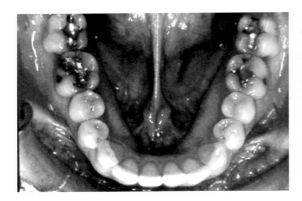
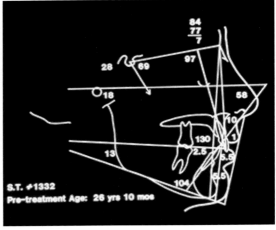

(*Continued*)

FIGURE 8–3   *(Continued)*

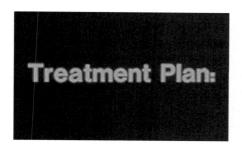

- **Rhinoplasty Discussed**

- **Rhinoplasty to Be Preformed Prior to Further Orthodontics**

- **Surgery:**

  Maxillary: 3 Piece Osteotomy

  Mandibular: Advancement

Porcelain Laminate Bonding of Maxillary Anteriors

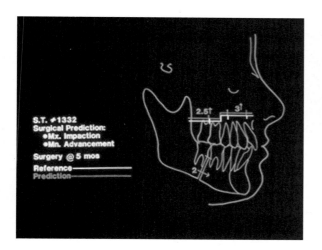

Total Treatment Time: 9 mos.

Finishing and Retention Procedures for Improved Aesthetics and Stability

Bjorn U. Zachrisson

INTRODUCTION

This chapter covers some aspects of aesthetics and stability in orthodontic fixed-appliance edgewise treatment. The following topics are considered:

1. Positioning of teeth in finishing.
2. Short- and long-term experiences with different types of intentional modifications of tooth morphology for cosmetic finishing purposes.
3. Differential retention with bonded retainers.

Supplementary information related to this chapter may be found in several of my recent publications.[1–9]

POSITIONING OF TEETH IN FINISHING

In my experience, the relationships of the contact points between neighboring teeth play an important role in the achievement of long-term stability. Both in orthodontically treated[10] and untreated teeth,[11] broken contact points may indicate predilection areas for further crowding or relapse. Unintentional undercorrection of malocclusions (so-called 9/10 orthodontics) may occur if careful study of pretreatment study models is not undertaken throughout and particularly toward the end of treatment.[1,2] This process may be summarized by our statement, "Look at the teeth— *not* at the archwires!" In my philosophy, the use of individualized arch-wires with built-in overcorrection (so-called 11/10 orthodontics) most eas-ily fulfills treatment objectives.[1,2] In addition to in-out positions and rotations of the incisors, axial inclination, torque, and marginal ridge heights are important factors that must be considered in treatment.

In-out positions and torque requirements in difficult treatment situa-tions are discussed in the following sections. Positioning of the teeth when maxillary lateral incisors are missing will be used as the model.

BUCCOLINGUAL WIDTH OF MAXILLARY CANINES AS REPLACEMENT FOR MISSING LATERAL INCISORS

With agenesis of lateral incisors and orthodontic space closure it is neces-sary to address the fact that the canines are wider buccolingually than the lateral incisors. This factor becomes more important the deeper the bite is pretreatment. If the width discrepancy is not addressed, the immediate results may be considered satisfactory, but even a slight reappearance of the deep overbite may lead to undesirable positions of recontoured canines. Figure 9–1 illustrates such a case. Either lingual grinding of the canine or positioning of this tooth more labially would probably have led to a better long-term result than was achieved in this case.

CLINICAL CROWN TORQUE

Clinical crown-root angulation and torque of maxillary canines may vary from patient to patient and within the same patient between the right and left sides (Fig. 9–3). Therefore, pretreatment evaluation of the crown torque is important when canines are to be moved mesially. Since the canines normally have more crown torque than the lateral incisors, and since frequently the first premolars may also have an inward tilt, a com-mon mistake in space closure of cases with missing lateral incisors is to undertorque the maxillary anterior teeth. Figure 9–2 illustrates such a case. Even though the positions of individual teeth except for the torque is good, the aesthetic result is not satisfactory. Thus, when looking at the patient, one gets the impression that all anterior teeth are tilting inward.

The situation may be even more complicated when there is bilateral agenesis of the maxillary lateral incisors and the clinical crown torque of the canines differs between the right and left sides (Fig. 9–3). In these sit-uations, which are not unusual, individual torque must be applied, or brackets with different torque values may be used on the right and left canines.

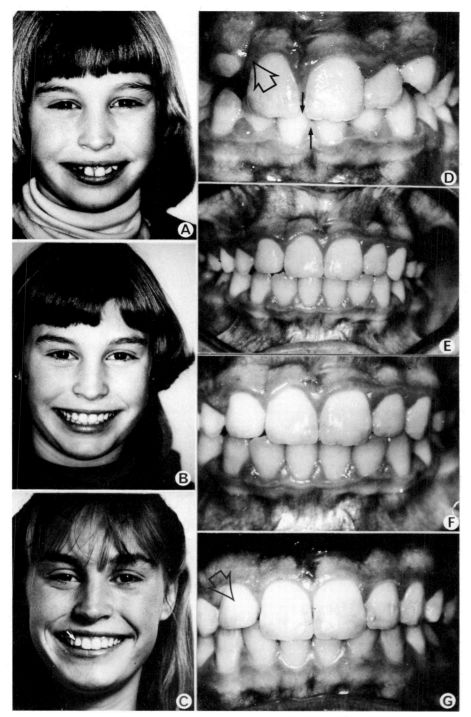

FIGURE 9–1 Young girl with congenitally missing maxillary right lateral incisor before (*A, D*), after (*B, E–F*), and seven years after orthodontic treatment (*C, G*). Note the deep overbite and midline deviation before therapy was instituted (*D*). After overbite correction, the ground canine on the right side and the intact lateral incisor on the left side were on the same level (*E–F*). Because of the buccolingual width difference between these teeth, however, the long-term result is not satisfactory. Thus, the right canine in lateral incisor position points outward with the settling of the deep overbite (arrows in *C, G*).

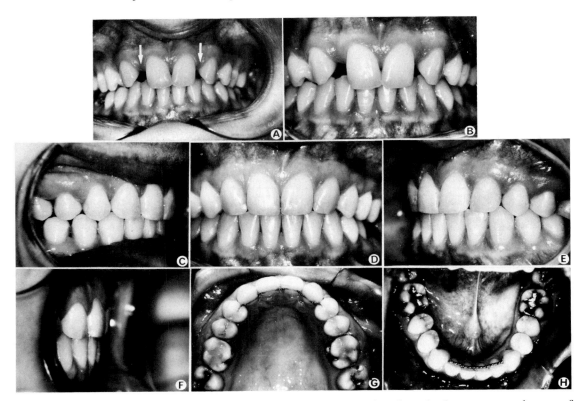

FIGURE 9–2   A common mistake associated with orthodontic space closure of patients with bilaterally missing maxillary lateral incisors is undertorque of the upper anterior region. Because the clinical crown of maxillary canines is generally tilted more lingually than that of most lateral incisors (see Fig. 9–3C), such canines need much lingual root torque when moved mesially (A, B). This case, although otherwise reasonably well treated (C–H), illustrates inadequate lingual root torque of both the central incisors (C, E–F) and the canines, which occupy the lateral incisor positions (D), making the aesthetic result unsatisfactory.

COSMETIC FINISHING

The following aspects of cosmetic finishing are addressed:

1. Grinding of teeth (incisal, labial, and lingual)
2. Mesiodistal enamel reduction in anterior and posterior regions.
3. Composite build-ups.
4. Gingivectomy to increase clinical crown length.

REMODELING OF THE TEETH BY GRINDING

Short-term results were published by Zachrisson and Mjör[12] in 1975. At that time clinical experiences with extensive recontouring of canines to

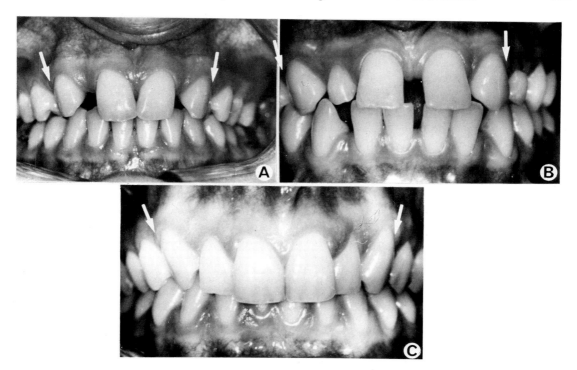

FIGURE 9–3 Three different cases, each illustrating marked differences in clinical crown torque between the right and left maxillary canines in the same patient (approximate crown angulation is indicated by the white arrows).

lateral incisors were supplemented with histological and radiographic findings. It was concluded that grinding may be done uneventfully provided abundant water spray is used and smooth and self-cleansing surfaces are prepared. Water cooling has the additional beneficial effect of reducing the pain associated with the grinding, thus eliminating the need for an anesthetic even in sensitive patients.

More recently, long-term results of grinding have become available. Thus, Thordarsson, Zachrisson, and Mjör[5] examined 26 patients (14 boys, 12 girls) about 10 years postgrinding in cases where canines had been recontoured to lateral incisors. Fifteen cases were treated unilaterally, 18 were bilaterally ground, and 4 comprised grinding of mandibular canines. The clinical examination at follow-up consisted of registration of color, mobility, percussion sensitivity, and sensitivity to hot and cold; electric pulp testing; and photograpic, radiographic, and SEM and stereomicroscopic study of epoxy resin replicas of the ground teeth. The results were favorable. There was no systematic difference in electric pulp response between ground and nonground canines. Color change was observed in 1 out of 37 teeth, and radiographic obliteration of crown or pulp canal was seen in only 2 of the 37 ground canines when compared with intact contralateral nonground canines.

In all of these instances, the procedure described earlier consisting of water cooling and preparation of smooth surfaces[12] was used. Figure 9–4 shows the instrumentation, including an inverted cone with diamond particles on the flat surface and a large round diamond for the lingual contouring. As shown in Figure 9–5, archwire bends in these cases called for some extrusion and labial movement of the canines. Again, the relationships of the contact points determined the size of the step bends that were required to position the canines in good sites. Figure 9–6 shows one of the unilateral cases before and after the orthodontic correction. This case was favored by good crown torque of the right canine pretreatment and an overbite that was not deep to start with.

The concepts of incisal adjustment for aesthetic improvement and for correction after contact of maxillary incisors with ceramic brackets will be considered in the oral presentation. For space reasons these topics are

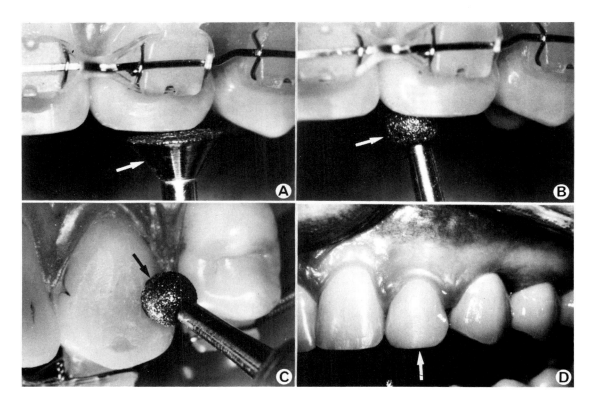

FIGURE 9–4   Instrumentation for grinding of maxillary canines that are to occupy the lateral incisor positions. An inverted cone with medium grit diamond particles on the flat surface (e.g., Horico number 022-055 or Komet number 810) is useful for the incisal cusp grinding (*A*), whereas a large round diamond is more useful for the lingual contouring (*B, C*). *D* shows final result of the same case as in Figures. 3*B* and 5.

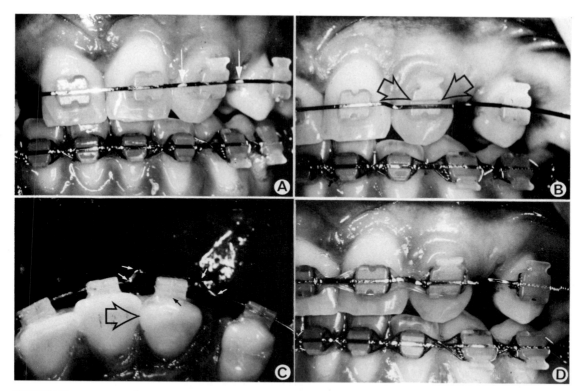

FIGURE 9–5   Archwire step bends when maxillary canines replace lateral incisors may include extrusion (*B*) to allow for cuspal grinding and also buccal movement (*C*). The contact point between the left central incisor and the canine is obviously undercorrected in *C* (open arrow). Marked step-out bends may be required (white arrows), particularly when thick ceramic brackets (black arrow) are used.

not elaborated upon in this text, and the reader is referred to other sources.[1,2] The same applies to the information on anterior and posterior stripping of teeth,[1,2,5] which will be analyzed from space requirement and aesthetic points of view. In particular, the possibility of normalizing abnormal tooth shapes and forms are discussed, and emphasis is given to reduction of interdental gingival recession and marginal opening up of triangular spaces between teeth.[12] Such spaces are commonly seen in adults after anterior crowding is relieved. It is recommended that the practitioner discuss with the patient before treatment the development of gingival triangles in order to avoid problems later.

When it comes to composite build-ups, some examples of correct and incorrect procedures are presented using premolar transplants to the anterior region as a model. Further information may be found in other publications of ours.[1,2,7,9]

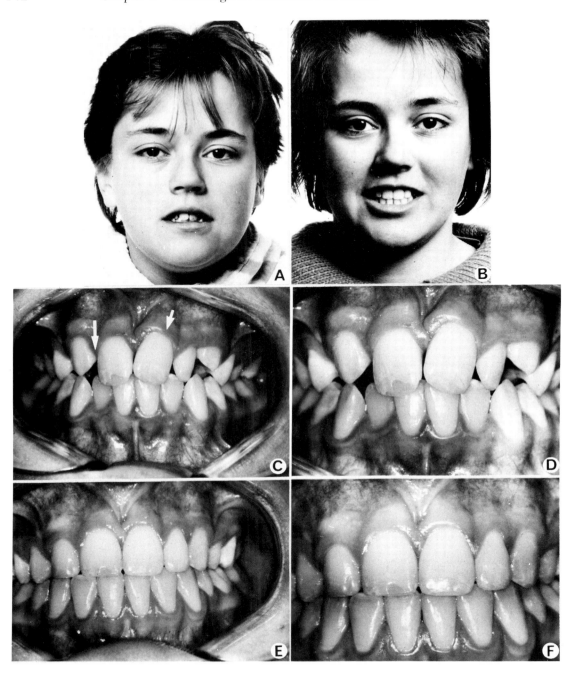

FIGURE 9–6 Young girl with agenesis of maxillary right lateral incisor before (*A, C–D*) and after orthodontic correction (*B, E–F*). Since the overbite was not deep to start with, and the clinical crown torque of the maxillary right canine is favorable for mesial movement, the long-term prognosis for this case is better than for the case in Figure 9–1. Also note the correction of the axial inclination of the maxillary left central incisor (arrow in *C*).

GINGIVECTOMY

Subsequent to our first report on gingivectomy to adjust clinical crown length[13] in 1977, this procedure has become a routine operation in Scandinavia. A useful modification for *adults* is illustrated here. As shown in Figure 9–7, the gingivectomy cut is limited in extent mesiodistally in order not to risk interdental recession. The procedure can be used on one or several teeth whenever an increase in clinical crown length is desirable from an aesthetic point of view (Fig. 9–7). As a rule, the gingiva heals by coronal proliferation, but this occurs only to 50–60 percent of the original gingival level.[13] Therefore, more tissue must be excised in the gingivectomy than the expected crown length increase.

Excellent oral hygiene is required for a period of four to six weeks after the surgery. It is important to alert the patient about toothbrushing damage. Gingival recession may occur after the removal of fixed appliances as a result of overzealous brushing. As a rule, most if not all adult patients need reinstruction in toothbrushing so as not to cause gingival recession and wedge-shaped tooth defects.

RETENTION

Several previous publications have discussed our preference for the use of different removable plates and bonded retainers according to the differential-retention principle.[1–4,6,8,14] Discussed here are (1) the present technique for bonding the thick (0.032 inches) and thin (0.0215 inches) spiral wire retainers; (2) new data on success rates of flexible spiral wire retainers; (3) modifications for deep-overbite situations; and (4) some aspects of repair of loose or broken retainers.

BONDING TECHNIQUE

The rigid spiral wire retainer (RSW) is made of 0.032-inch spiral wire.* The lingual saliva ejector † is ideal for providing a dry working field, with a 0.8–0.9-mm soft steel wire inserted in the tubing to facilitate handling. No lip expander is needed, but one or more cotton rolls may be inserted labially. Figure 9–8 illustrates how the wire is adjusted carefully to all four incisors and secured in place with two or three steel ties. Bonding is a two-step procedure, as before,[3] but trimming after handling the bulk of adhe-

---

*Unitek Corporation/3M, Monrovia, CA 91016-7118 (number 709-060).

†Unitek Corporation/3M Monrovia, CA 91016-7118 (number 709-040).

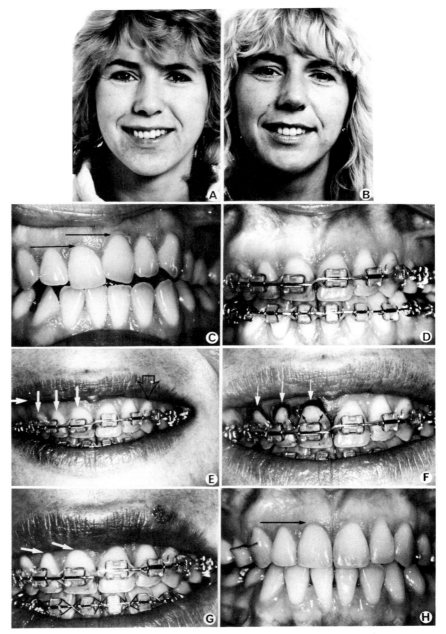

FIGURE 9–7   Modification of gingivectomy technique for adults. The asymmetric smile line before orthodontic therapy (*A, C*) indicated gingivectomy on the maxillary right side (canine through central incisor) at the end of treatment (*F*). As indicated by the arrows in *F*, the excision for adults may be limited in extent mesiodistally so as to avoid the occurrence of interdental gingival recession. Subsequent to the coronal regeneration, the marginal gingival levels are more even (*B, H*) and the healing takes place with preservation of nice interdental papillae (*H*). Note the improvement when comparing the marginal tissue levels in *C* and *H* and the smile lines in *E* and *G*.

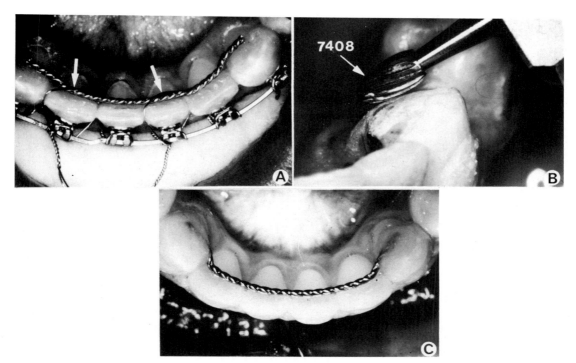

FIGURE 9–8   Technique for making and bonding the RSW 3 × 3 retainer. A 0.032-inch spiral wire is carefully adapted to the lingual surface of all four mandibular incisors and secured with two (or three) steel ligatures (arrows in *A*) while the fixed appliances remain in place. The steel tie on the left central incisor is turned clockwise, and the one on the right lateral incisor is turned counterclockwise. Trimming of the bulk of composite material (*B*) is made with a large tungsten-carbide bur (number 7408). Note that this type of retainer wire is bonded only on the terminal units (*C*).

sive is now done with a large oval tungsten-carbide bur (number 7408). This bur is ideal for giving optimal contour to the adhesive (Fig. 9–8).

The flexible spiral wire retainer (FSW) is made of 0.0215-inch five-stranded wire. The wire is adjusted to accurate stone models using three-prong pliers. It is bonded to all teeth in a segment. Figure 9–9 illustrates the new approach to safely ensure that the wire is bonded in optimal position. A four-handed approach is utilized for the initial tacking. Thus, while the orthodontist holds the wire in place by hand in the mouth (Figure 9–9*A*), an assistant adds a small amount of fast-setting composite to one of the central incisors (Fig. 9–9*B*). When set, the position of the wire can be checked carefully (Fig. 9–9*C*); if it is satisfactory, the orthodontist tacks the remaining teeth (Fig. 9–9*D*). The bulk is added next, and trimming is done with different tungsten-carbide burs (numbers 7006, 7408, and 2).

** Masel Orthodontics, Inc. Bristol, PA 19007-6892 (Penta-One).

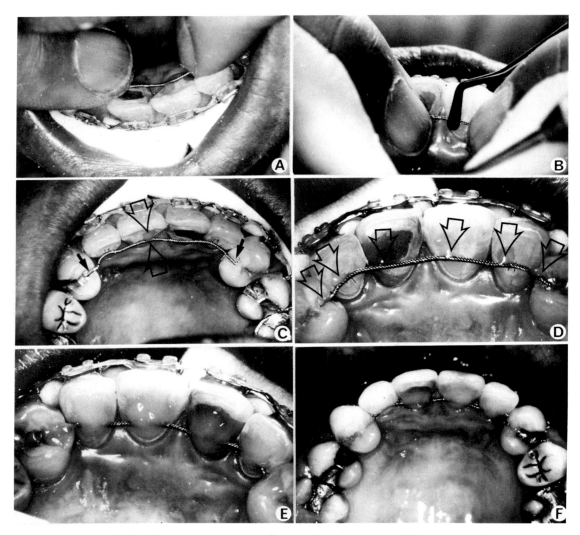

FIGURE 9–9   Technique for bonding a six-unit FSW retainer. To secure optimal position of the 0.0215-inch Penta-One wire, a four-handed approach for initial tacking has proved to be very useful (*A–C*). Small grooves were prepared in the occlusal surface of the first premolars in this case to help hold the rotation of the mesially moved premolars in canine positions (*C*).

While the orthodontist holds the retainer wire by hand, an assistant puts on the initial fast-setting composite on one incisor only (*A–C*). When the composite has set, a good impression of the fit and passiveness of the wire is obtained (*C*). If the impression is acceptable, the rest is more or less a filling-in procedure. The remaining teeth are tacked by the orthodontist (*D*), and bulk composite is added next (*E*). Note that this type of retainer wire is bonded to all teeth within a segment (*F*).

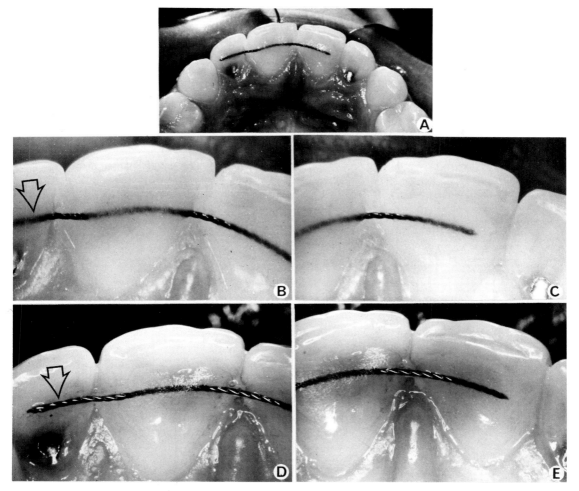

FIGURE 9–10   A thin FSW retainer bonded by the author in 1976. *A–C* shows the condition at time of bonding, and *D–E* illustrates the status 12 years later. Note the evident wear of the composite bonding material (compare the open arrow areas in *B* and *D*).

SUCCESS RATE OF BONDED FLEXIBLE SPIRAL WIRE RETAINERS

Over the past five or more years, our preferred wire size for the thin FSW retainer has been 0.0215 inches, in contrast to earlier[14] when thinner wire diameters were used. We now have accumulated data on the frequency of failures (loosening, wire fracture) with three-stranded (Rocky Mountain Tri-Flex, and GAC Wildcat) and five-stranded (Masel Penta-One) wires. This material is presented elsewhere by Dahl and Zachrisson.[6]

The observation time for 55 three-stranded wire retainers in the maxilla is 6.0 years on average (standard deviation 1.6), and for 29 retainers in the mandible it is 5.7 years (standard deviation 1.5). On average, the former contained 5.5 teeth (standard deviation 1.6) and the latter 6.7 teeth (standard deviation 1). Loosening occurred in 23.2 percent of the patients with the maxillary retainers and in 10.3 percent of those with the mandibular retainers. Most of the loose bonds occurred between the adhesive and the wire and happened in combination with wear of the adhesive. Figure 9–10 demonstrates the long-term status of an FSW retainer, with evident wear after more than 12 years in place in situ, although at this stage the retainer was still intact.

The failure rate just given corresponds to 9.5 percent of all 304 bonded teeth in the maxilla and 2 percent of the 148 bonded teeth in the mandible. Wire fracture occurred in 23.2 percent of the 56 patients with maxillary retainers, or 5.2 percent of the 249 interdental areas. In the mandible, the corresponding figures were 10.3 percent of patients, or 2.4 percent of 123 interdental areas. Most loosening occurred within the first year, whereas fatigue fracture occurred at irregular intervals throughout the study period.

Because of the high incidence of fracture, a *five*-stranded 0.0215-inch wire has been used exclusively since October 1986. Our study material with this wire consists of 64 maxillary retainers with an average observation period of 3.1 years (standard deviation 0.6) and 17 mandibular retainers with an observation period of 3.2 years (standard deviation 0.6). The failure rates in terms of loosening with the five-stranded wire were only 7.8 percent of the patients with the maxillary retainers and 5.9 percent of those with the mandibular retainers. Fracture occurred in only 3.1 percent of the patients with the maxillary retainers over the 3.1 years, which is encouraging.

DEEP-OVERBITE AND BONDED LINGUAL RETAINERS

Failure rates of 50 percent for periods of from 4 to 40 months were recently reported for FSW retainers by Årtun and Urbye.[15] Most of these patients had had marked periodontal breakdown, and some deep overbite remained after treatment. In our material[6] deep bites were generally corrected by orthodontic treatment, which in part may explain the difference in the rate of success. Clearly, the failure rate will increase if the patient bites on the retainer wire, which is bonded. Surprisingly, however, in some such instances the abrasion on the wire may be so heavy that the round wire is worn flat (Fig. 9–11). Due to the spirals in the wire, such bonds may still be intact for several years. But it is an advantage, of course, if direct impingement on the wire can be avoided. Figures 9–12 and 9–13 illustrate two different approaches to overcoming this problem. In Figure

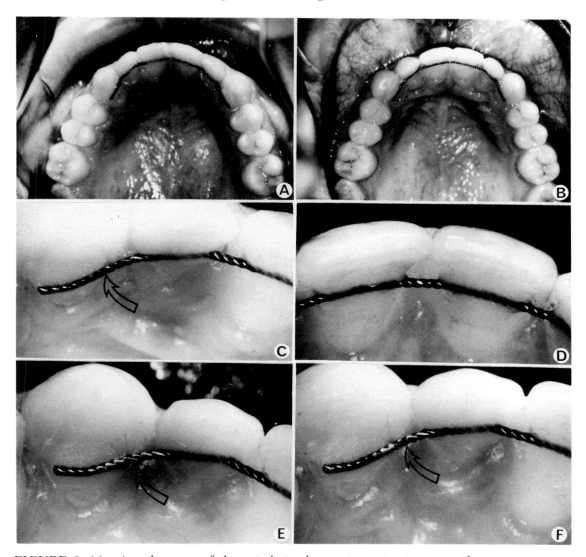

FIGURE 9–11 An advantage of the spirals in the retainer wire is to provide undercut areas for the bonding adhesive even though patients may bite directly on the adhesive and wire. This case illustrates the conditions at the time of bonding of an FSW retainer (*A*) and the situation seven years later (*B–F*). Note that the round spiral wire has actually become worn flat (open arrows in *C, E,* and *F*), but the retainer bonds are intact.

9–12 the wire was bonded as far gingivally as possible, whereas in Figure 9–13 small grooves were made in the enamel to partly hide the retainer wire. Figure 9–13*G–I* shows this retainer after 2.4 years and indicates wear of the composite and in one site a loosening between the enamel and the composite. Such failures are most likely due to moisture contamination during setting of the adhesive.[3]

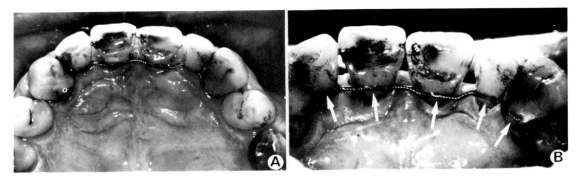

FIGURE 9–12   In compromise situations when some deep overbite remains posttreatment, the FSW retainer can be bonded as far gingivally as in this case.

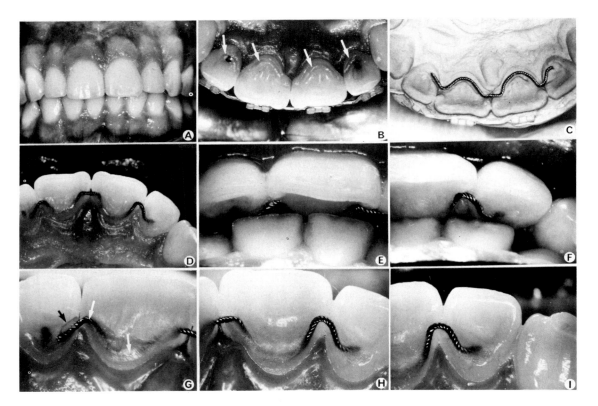

FIGURE 9–13   Another solution than in Figure 9–12 when a deep overbite remains after therapy (A) is to prepare small grooves in the enamel of the maxillary incisors (B–C). After careful adaptation of the thin retainer wire (C), it is bonded, as shown in Figure 9–9. E–F shows the condition at the time of bonding, whereas G–I illustrates the retainer status 2.4 years later. There is evident abrasive wear of the composite and even some flattening of the retainer wire (solid white arrows in G) and a bond failure between enamel and adhesive (black arrow).

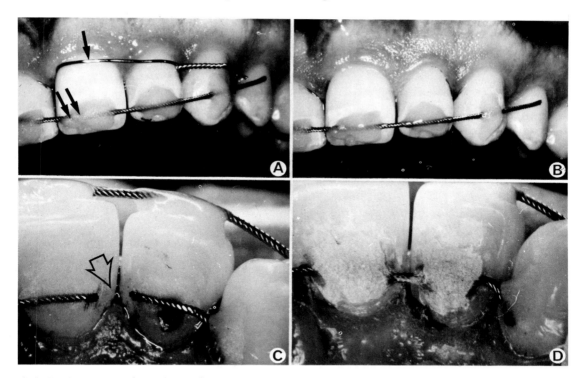

FIGURE 9–14   The repair of broken retainers may be instituted by moving loose teeth with the fingers or with ligatures. When in place, the steel tie is replaced with a temporary labial wire (double arrows in *A*). This will secure the totally undisturbed setting of the composite covering the repair wire on the lingual side (*C–D*). Immediately after setting of the adhesive, the labially bonded wire is removed.

REPAIR OF BONDED RETAINERS

Different forms of repair may be needed for broken or loosely bonded retainers. If discovered early, small relapses of teeth may frequently be directly corrected by moving the teeth with finger pressure, steel ligatures, or elastic ties, as the teeth are relatively mobile. Before repairing the lingual side, it has proved helpful to use a temporary labial wire, as indicated in Figure 9–14. The wire totally secures the undisturbed setting of the adhesive on the repair side because the wire prevents the teeth from moving. Immediately after repair, the labial retainer wire is removed.

SUMMARY

This chapter discussed finishing and retention in orthodontics in order to try to improve the aesthetics and stability of the treatment result. Emphasis was placed on aspects of tooth positioning, cosmetic remodeling of teeth in adults and children, and experiences with the use of thick (0.032-inch) and thin (0.0215-inch) spiral wire retainers bonded lingually to the teeth.

REFERENCES

1. Zachrisson BU: Excellence in finishing. Part I. J Clin Orthod 20:460–482, 1986.
2. Zachrisson BU: Excellence in finishing. Part II. J Clin Orthod 20:536–559, 1986.
3. Zachrisson BU: Bonding in orthodontics. *In* Graber TM, Swain BF: Orthodontics: Current Principles and Techniques. St. Louis, C. V. Mosby, 1985, pp. 485–563.
4. Zachrisson BU: The bonded lingual retainer and multiple spacing of anterior teeth. J Clin Orthod 17:838–846, 1983.
5. Thordarson A, Zachrisson BU, Mjör IA: Remodeling of canines to the shape of lateral incisors by grinding: A long-term clinical and radiographic evaluation. Am J Orthod 100:123–132, 1991.
6. Dahl E, Zachrisson BU: Long-term experience with direct-bonded lingual retainers. J Clin Orthod 25:619–630, 1991.
7. Paulsen HU, Zachrisson BU: Autotransplantation of teeth and orthodontic treatment planning. *In* Andreasen JO: Atlas of Replantation and Transplantation of Teeth. Mediglobe SA, Fribourg, Switzerland, Ch.10, pp. 257–276, 1992.
8. Axelsson S, Zachrisson BU: Clinical experience with direct-bonded labial retainers. J Clin Orthod 26:480–490, 1992.
9. Stenvik A, Zachrisson BU: Orthodontic closure and transplantation in the treatment of missing anterior teeth. An overview. Endodont Dent Traumatol 9:1993 (in press).
10. Little RM, Wallen TR, Riedel RR: Stability and relapse of mandibular anterior alignment—First premolar extraction cases treated by traditional edgewise orthodontics. Am J Orthod 80:349–365, 1981.
11. Humerfeldt A, Slagsvold O: Changes in occlusion and craniofacial pattern between 11 and 25 years of age. A follow-up study of individuals with normal occlusion. Trans Eur Orthod Soc 113–122, 1972.
12. Zachrisson BU, Mjör IA. Remodelling of teeth by grinding. Am J Orthod 68:545–553, 1975.
13. Monefeldt I, Zachrisson BU: Adjustment of clinical crown height by gingivectomy following orthodontic space closure. Am J Orthod 47:256–264, 1977.
14. Zachrisson BU: Clinical experience with direct-bonded orthodontic retainers. Am J Orthod 71:440–448, 1977.
15. Årtun J, Urbye KS: The effect of orthodontic treatment on periodontal bone support in patients with advanced loss of marginal periodontium. Am J Orthod 93:143–148, 1988.
16. Gaare D, Rölla G, Aryadi FJ, Ouderaa Fvd: Improvement of gingival health by toothbrushing in individuals with large amounts of calculus. J Clin Period 17:38–41, 1990.

The Long-Term Stability of Orthognathic Surgery

Peter M. Sinclair

INTRODUCTION

The advent of orthognathic surgery has given the practicing orthodontist, in conjunction with the oral surgeon, the ability to correct skeletal deformities that had previously been camouflaged by orthodontics alone. Often these orthodontic treatment results were unsatisfactory since they required severe dental compensations to accommodate the poor skeletal relationship. With the recent advances in orthognathic surgery, however, it has become possible for the surgeon to address many deformities that were previously untreatable. Long-term stability following these surgical procedures has been of major concern since the early days of orthognathic surgery because the final long-term result, both aesthetic and functional, is directly related to the postsurgical stability.

The early studies of mandibular advancements[1,2] and maxillary LeFort I osteotomies[3] revealed that mandibular relapse tended to be greater than maxillary relapse. Therefore, many studies of stability in the 1970s concentrated on mandibular advancements utilizing follow-up cephalometric radiographs in an attempt to identify the relapse patterns and their etiology.[4–6] These studies, as well as studies in the early 1980s by Schendel and Epker[7] and by Lake et al[8] demonstrated that relapse primarily occurred during intermaxillary fixation and immediately following the release of fixation, so that the long-term results were not always predictable. Some studies of the relapse patterns following maxillary LeFort I osteotomies were also reported during this period[9,10] and demonstrated greater overall stability than seen for mandibular advancements, but documented instances of instability for individual patients. In the late 1970s further advances in surgical techniques allowed surgical procedures to be performed simultaneously in both the maxilla and the mandible. Early studies of double jaw surgery reported lesser amounts of mandibular relapse and greater maxillary relapse than for single jaw procedures performed independently.[11]

Numerous theories regarding the primary etiologic causes of relapse have been advanced and studied. These include (1) stretching of the muscles of mastication and the suprahyoid musculature,[2,12] (2) condylar distraction during surgery,[7,13,14] (3) counterclockwise rotation of the mandible,[1,12,15] and (4) rotational position changes between the proximal and distal segments.[8,16]

Simultaneously, various surgical techniques and postsurgical therapies were advocated in order to minimize relapse, and numerous studies were conducted to evaluate their results. These techniques included suprahyoid myotomies[15,17,18] and cervical collars utilized to reduce muscle tension following surgery.[1,2,11]

Numerous fixation techniques have been advocated to reduce relapse postsurgically. These have included (1) upper and lower border wiring of the mandible,[19] (2) Steinmann pins to stabilize the maxilla,[20] (3) skeletal wire fixation,[7] and (4) rigid fixation.[21] Recently, studies involving isolated mandibular advancements[22,23] and maxillary LeFort I procedures[24] have indicated a strong potential for reduced relapse using the two most popular of these alternate techniques: skeletal wire fixation and rigid fixation.

Although numerous papers have been published evaluating the stability of the major surgical procedures (i.e., sagittal split, LeFort I osteotomy), no clear picture has as yet emerged as to their overall long-term stability.

Most of the studies on stability have concentrated their evaluations on the short-term (i.e., the first six to eight weeks) postsurgical period. Few studies have evaluated relapse out to one year postsurgery. Among those who have examined stability at one year postsurgery, many have used small sample sizes with heterogeneous groups, often including patients with clefts or other congenital deformities. In addition, the fact that different surgical procedures were frequently carried out on patients in the same sample has further reduced our ability to evaluate long-term results.

Therefore, the purpose of this chapter is to review current knowledge of the long-term (defined in this chapter as one year postsurgery) stability of the most commonly performed single and double jaw orthognathic procedures. In most cases only papers with reasonably large (N = 20) homogeneous samples, where the data for three time periods was clearly identifiable, are discussed.

DATA ORGANIZATION

These time periods are as follows:

1. T_1 to T_2:   Initial to postsurgery.
2. T_2 to T_3:   Postsurgery to 6–8 weeks.
3. T_3 to T_4:   6–8 weeks to 1 year.

In the figures that follow, the tabular data are presented using these three time periods, with positive (+) signs indicating changes in either the anterior or superior direction and negative (−) signs indicating changes in either the posterior or inferior direction. When presented graphically the data appear as though one is viewing a cephalometric tracing facing to the right. The arrow starting at the origin (i.e., zero mm) represents the amount and direction of the surgical change. The second and third arrows reflect the amount and direction of the short-term (T_2–T_3) and long-term (T_3–T_4) postsurgical changes, respectively. The percentage value represents the total percentage relapse seen after one year.

For purposes of simplicity and clarity only mandibular changes at B-point and maxillary changes at A-point are evaluated. Similarly, the discussion also focuses on the primary direction of surgical change while recognizing that rotational changes and changes in other directions are likely to influence the changes seen in the principal direction.

MANDIBULAR ADVANCEMENT

WIRE FIXATION (Fig. 10–1)

Using the well-conducted Lake (1981) study[8] as a baseline, one sees that there was 1.6 mm of posterior relapse during fixation and little change from eight weeks out to one year. Kohn in 1978,[6] with a larger mandibular advancement while seeing a similar amount of short-term relapse, also encountered a considerable amount of long-term relapse. The total relapse seen over one year in these two studies (24 percent and 38 percent) is reflective of many studies carried out during this period that utilized only interdental wiring for fixation. As reflected by the changes seen in the Sandor study (1984),[25] when skeletal fixation using circumzygomatic and circummandibular wires was utilized the amount of relapse seen was considerably smaller. Recently, Watske[26] has noted a different pattern of changes, with the initial posterior relapse being almost counterbalanced by a long-term forward movement, thus producing only a small (6 percent) net relapse. Whether this pattern will be found in other contemporary studies or is due to some specific feature of the surgical technique remains to be determined.

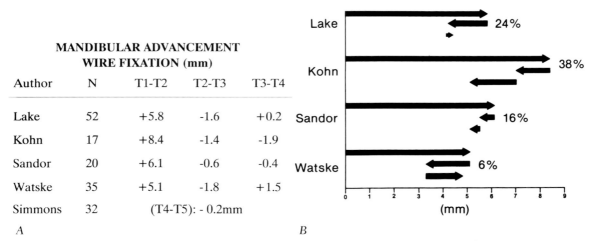

MANDIBULAR ADVANCEMENT
WIRE FIXATION (mm)

Author	N	T1-T2	T2-T3	T3-T4
Lake	52	+5.8	-1.6	+0.2
Kohn	17	+8.4	-1.4	-1.9
Sandor	20	+6.1	-0.6	-0.4
Watske	35	+5.1	-1.8	+1.5
Simmons	32	(T4-T5): - 0.2mm		

A   *B*

FIGURE 10–1   Tabular (*A*) and graphic (*B*) representations of the changes during and after mandibular advancement with wire fixation as measured at B-point.

In one of the few studies to evaluate mandibular stability beyond one year, Simmons[27] noted only minimal changes from T_4 (one year) out to T_5 (five years). Further studies of this duration are required to provide a truly good long-term appreciation of mandibular stability.

RIGID FIXATION (Fig. 10–2)

When comparing the stability of mandibular advancement with rigid fixation to that of wire fixation some differences are immediately apparent.[26,28–30] Of prime importance is the finding that the net changes for the rigid studies are in an anterior direction rather than in the posterior direction previously noted for the wire fixation samples. The magnitude of the relapse is less than half of that seen with the earlier interdental wire fixation studies, but it is only moderately better than the contemporary skeletal wire fixation studies.

However, when the incidence of relapse in Watske's matched samples of contemporary skeletal wire and rigid fixation groups are compared some interesting findings emerge. During the first six weeks following surgery (Fig. 10–3) approximately 40 percent of the wire fixation sample demonstrated between 2 and 4 mm of posterior relapse. An additional 5 percent showed greater than 4 mm of posterior relapse, whereas a similar number underwent 2–4 mm of anterior relapse. Thus, approximately 50 percent of the wire fixation sample demonstrated instability during fixation, with the preponderance of change being in the posterior direction. In contrast, only 25 percent of the rigid sample demonstrated significant

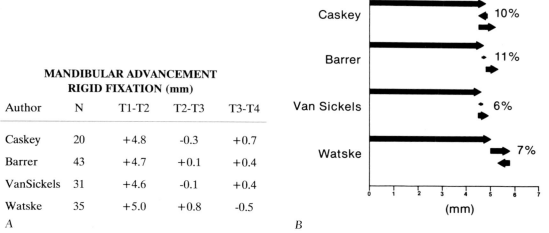

MANDIBULAR ADVANCEMENT RIGID FIXATION (mm)				
Author	N	T1-T2	T2-T3	T3-T4
Caskey	20	+4.8	-0.3	+0.7
Barrer	43	+4.7	+0.1	+0.4
VanSickels	31	+4.6	-0.1	+0.4
Watske	35	+5.0	+0.8	-0.5

A   B

FIGURE 10–2   Tabular (A) and graphic (B) representations of the changes during and after mandibular advancement with rigid fixation as measured at B-point.

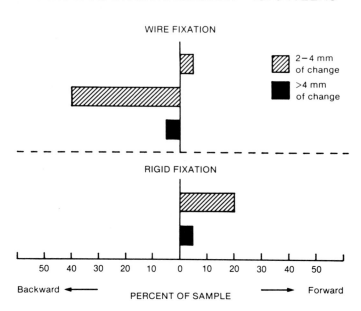

FIGURE 10–3   The incidence of relapse in Watske's rigid and wire fixation samples over the first six weeks postsurgery.

relapse, with most of the changes being between 2 and 4 mm in an anterior direction.

From six weeks to one year (Fig. 10–4) somewhat different findings were noted. About 40 percent of the wire fixation sample now demonstrated a tendency to come forward whereas in the rigid sample 25 percent of the cases continued to come forward and 20 percent were moving posteriorly.

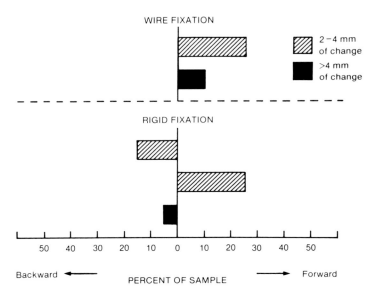

FIGURE 10–4   The incidence of relapse in Watske's rigid and wire fixation samples from six weeks to one year post-surgery.

MANDIBULAR SETBACK (Fig. 10–5)

The vast majority of studies evaluating mandibular setbacks have utilized wire fixation. The studies reviewed in this chapter (Fig. 10–5) can be conveniently divided into three pairs. First, Kobayashi[31] and Rosenquist,[32] with moderate setbacks of 5.4 and 8.4 mm, noted 18 percent and 22 percent, respectively, of anterior relapse after one year. Forward movement was seen during both the short-and long-term periods and totaled between 1.2 and 1.5 mm. In contrast, Astrand[33] and Vijayaraghavan[34] reported considerably larger mean setbacks and noted anterior relapse of 2.4 and 3.1 mm, respectively, after one year. This greater absolute amount of relapse translated into 20 percent and 31 percent net change for the two studies and is reflective of many studies suggesting that larger setbacks are more likely to undergo greater postsurgical changes.

Recently Phillips et al[35] compared skeletal stability following sagittal split and transoral vertical ramus osteotomies (TOVROs). Their findings indicated different patterns of relapse, with the SSs coming forward postsurgery whereas the TOVROs showed continued posterior change. Also of note was the fact that the relapse seen in the SSs (38 percent of the surgical change) was considerably greater than that seen for the TOVROs (23 percent of the surgical change).

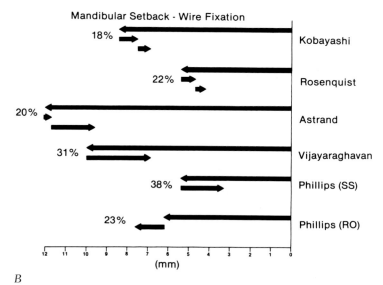

MANDIBULAR SETBACK WIRE FIXATION (mm)				
Author	N	T1-T2	T2-T3	T3-T4
Kobayashi	34	-8.4	+0.9	+0.6
Rosenquist	14	-5.4	+0.7	+0.5
Astrand	35	-12.0	+0.3	+2.1
Vijayar- aghavan	16	-10.0	-	+3.1
Phillips (SS)	19	-5.4	-	+2.1
Phillips (RO)	20	-6.2	-	-1.4

A

B

FIGURE 10–5 Tabular (*A*) and graphic (*B*) representations of the changes during and after mandibular setback with wire fixation as measured at B-point.

Unfortunately, comparison with setbacks carried out with rigid fixation is not possible due to the lack of studies of this type. Of note, however, is the study by Franco et al,[36] in which, with a sample of 14 patients, the researchers showed an average of 2.1 mm, or 43 percent, anterior relapse following a mean of 4.9 mm of surgical setback. Whether or not future studies confirm this finding or this finding is found to be reflective of early experiences with rigid fixation remains to be seen.

FACTORS INFLUENCING MANDIBULAR STABILITY

Since the early days of orthognathic surgery it has been hypothesized that the greater the amount of mandibular surgical movement, the greater the relapse. Although reported numerous times in case studies and generally accepted to be true, little scientific data are available to confirm this concept. For his mandibular advancements using wire fixation, Lake[8] noted a correlation of r = 0.60 between the magnitude of advancement and the relapse over one year, while Van Sickels[30] demonstrated a similar correlation (r = 0.62) with a rigid fixation sample. In general, both of these authors as well as many others have felt that advancements greater than 10 mm showed less stability and that factors such as a high mandibular plane angle and poor proximal segment control during surgery were significant predisposing factors to increased mandibular instability.

In her evaluation of the two techniques for mandibular setback, Phillips[35] noted that the sagittal split group showed a somewhat higher correlation (r = 0.65) between the magnitude of surgical change and relapse than did the TOVRO group (r = 0.56). In general, considerably more investigation of these interactions appears to be necessary to allow for the identification and possible future control of factors likely to precipitate mandibular instability.

MAXILLARY IMPACTION

WIRE FIXATION (Fig. 10–6)

Several long-term studies have evaluated maxillary impaction when carried out as a single, independent procedure. Overall, they demonstrate a net tendency for continued superior settling following surgery. Whereas

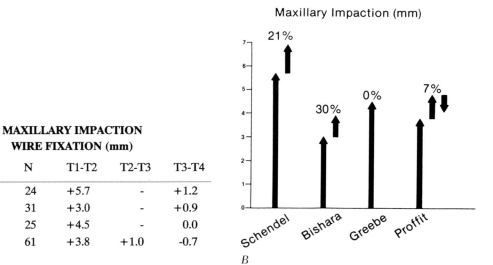

MAXILLARY IMPACTION
WIRE FIXATION (mm)

Author	N	T1-T2	T2-T3	T3-T4
Schendel	24	+5.7	-	+1.2
Bishara	31	+3.0	-	+0.9
Greebe	25	+4.5	-	0.0
Proffit	61	+3.8	+1.0	-0.7

A   *B*

FIGURE 10–6   Tabular (*A*) and graphic (*B*) representations of the changes during and after isolated maxillary impaction with wire fixation as measured at A-point.

MAXILLA UP —
VERTICAL CHANGES

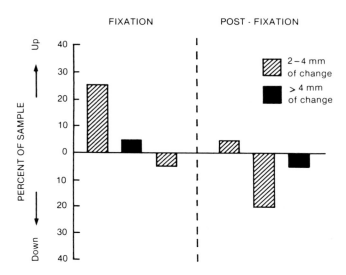

FIGURE 10–7 The incidence of relapse in Proffit's wire fixation maxillary impaction sample as measured at A-point.

some studies suggest minimal long-term change (Greebe 0 percent,[37] Proffit 7 percent[38]), others reflect a significant degree of relapse (Schendel 21 percent,[9] Bishara 30 percent[39]), although the actual amounts are quite small—often around only 1 mm.

In Proffit's[38] sample it is interesting to note that the direction of postoperative change was quite different in the short- and the long-term periods (Fig. 10–7). During the fixation period, 25 percent of the sample demonstrated superior movements between 2 and 4 mm, with an additional 5 percent showing greater than 4 mm of superior movement. In contrast, about 5 percent of the sample moved inferiorly during this period. Postfixation the picture was reversed, with 20 percent of the sample showing moderate amounts (2–4 mm) of inferior movement, 5 percent showing greater than 4 mm of inferior movement, and 5 percent continuing to move superiorly. Thus, about 30 percent of this sample continued to show relapse at A-point out to one year following surgery. Proffit also noted that posterior maxillary stability was somewhat better, with only half as many cases showing significant postsurgical changes.

When single versus multiple segment maxillary impactions with wire fixation were compared by Proffit,[38] little difference was found between their long-term stability (Fig. 10–8). Both groups showed continued superior settling in the short term followed by long-term inferior movement,

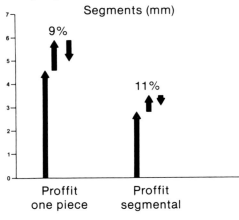

MAXILLARY IMPACTION
WIRE FIXATION (mm)

Author	N	T1-T2	T2-T3	T3-T4
Proffit /one piece	36	+4.6	+1.3	-0.9
Proffit /segmented	25	+2.8	+0.7	-0.4

A

B

FIGURE 10–8   Tabular (*A*) and graphic (*B*) representations of the changes during and after one-piece and segmental maxillary impactions.

MAXILLARY IMPACTION
and
MANDIBULAR ADVANCEMENT

Author	N	T1-T2	T2-T3	T3-T4
Bramer	12	A-(V) +3.1	-	-0.4
Turvey	53	A-(V) +3.0	-	-0.5
Satrom	9	A-(V) +2.2	-	-0.8

WIRE FIXATION (mm)

A

MAXILLARY IMPACTION
and
MANDIBULAR ADVANCEMENT

Author	N	T1-T2	T2-T3	T3-T4
Hennes	24	A-(V) +4.3	-	-0.1
Satrom	26	A-(V) +2.5	-	-0.1

RIGID FIXATION (mm)

B

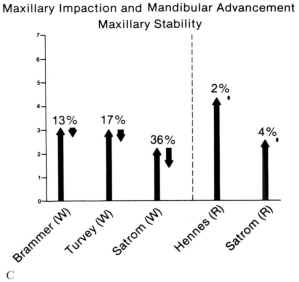

C

FIGURE 10–9   *A*, Tabular representation of the vertical maxillary changes as measured at A-point in the wire fixation studies. *B*, Tabular representation of the vertical maxillary changes as measured at A-point in the rigid fixation studies. *C*, Graphic representation of the vertical maxillary changes as measured at A-point for the wire (W) and rigid (R) studies.

resulting in a net of less than $1/2$ mm of long-term superior relapse. This produced overall relapse percentages of 9 percent for the one-piece maxillas and 11 percent for the segmental procedures—values comparable to those of the studies described previously.[7,39]

MAXILLARY IMPACTION AND MANDIBULAR ADVANCEMENT

VERTICAL MAXILLARY CHANGES

When maxillary impaction is carried out as part of a simultaneous double jaw procedure a different pattern of relapse is found than that previously seen in isolated maxillary impactions. In the wire fixation studies[11,40,41] (Fig. 10–9) there was a small but consistent tendency for the maxilla to move inferiorly following surgery. These changes were well under 1 mm and ranged from 13 percent up to 36 percent of the surgical change. Stability in the rigid fixation sample[41,42] was even better, with minimal (2 percent and 4 percent) postoperative inferior movement being noted. Although these samples are small, they might be taken to suggest that maxillary stability in double jaw cases, particularly when rigid fixation is used, is certainly no worse—and perhaps even a little better—than when maxillary surgery alone is performed.

ANTEROPOSTERIOR MANDIBULAR CHANGES (FIG. 10–10)

The data from the group of three studies in which the patients underwent mandibular advancement with wire fixation as part of a double jaw procedure[11,40,41] provides an interesting comparison to the isolated mandibular advancements described previously (Fig. 10–1).[6,8,25,26] Although they underwent considerably larger advancements (probably due to the greater severity of the malocclusions in the cases warranting double jaw surgery), both the average amount of posterior relapse (1.4 mm) and the overall relapse percentages were very similar to those found in the isolated mandibular advancement studies. In fact, the mandibular stability seen in the double jaw rigid fixation studies[41,42] appeared to be superior to that seen in the isolated rigid fixation mandibular advancements (Fig. 10–2).[26,28–30]

MAXILLARY ADVANCEMENT (Fig. 10–11)

Quantifiable data for maxillary advancements are conspicuously lacking in the current literature, particularly where long-term evaluations are concerned. In the two wire fixation studies available,[43,44] long-term posterior

MAXILLARY IMPACTION
and
MANDIBULAR ADVANCEMENT

Author	N	T1-T2	T2-T3	T3-T4
Brammer	12(W)	+12.8	-	-1.8
Turvey	53(W)	+8.5	-	-0.6
Satrom	9(W)	+7.1	-	-1.9
Hennes	24(R)	+10.3	-	+0.1
Satrom	26(R)	+8.6	-	-0.5

MANDIBULAR STABILITY (mm)

A

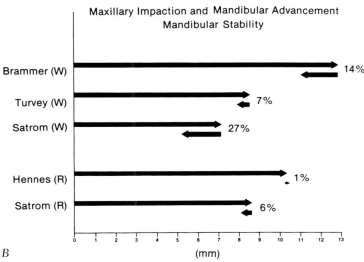

B

FIGURE 10–10 Tabular (*A*) and graphic (*B*) representations of the anteroposterior mandibular changes seen in double jaw surgery.

relapse ranged from a total of 0.5 mm to 1 mm, representing 7 percent and 20 percent of the surgical change, respectively. When rigid fixation is used the data appear to be similar, with a moderate amount of posterior relapse being seen.[44,45] With the small samples available it is difficult to reach any definitive conclusions, particularly when the confounding factors of different types of grafting procedures (i.e., bone versus hydroxylapatite) used in the various studies are included. Of interest, however, is a comparison between Weiss's[44] two samples, both operated in the same fashion, which while being somewhat different during the fixation period, show little long-term difference.

MAXILLARY DOWNGRAFT (Fig. 10–12)

Historically, maxillary downgraft has been one of the least stable orthognathic procedures; current long-term data (unfortunately only six months

MAXILLARY ADVANCEMENT

Author	N	T1-T2	T2-T3	T3-T4
Teuscher	16(W)	+7.1	-0.4	-0.1
Weiss	24(W)	+4.6	-0.1	-0.9
Wardrop	10(R)	+5.8	-	-0.4
Weiss	14(R)	+4.8	+0.4	-1.2

A

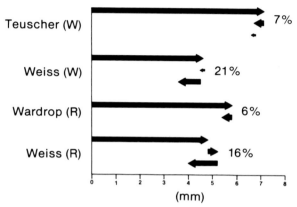

FIGURE 10–11   Tabular (*A*) and graphic (*B*) representations of the changes during and after maxillary advancement.

B

MAXILLARY DOWNGRAFT

Author	N	T1-T2	T2-T3	T3-T4
Hedemark	15(W)	-3.2	-	+2.5 (6m)
Bell	13(W)	-6.8	-	+1.9 (6m)
Quejada	10(R)	-8.9	+1.1	+1.0 (6m)
Persson	16(R)	-6.6	+1.5	0.0 (6m)

A

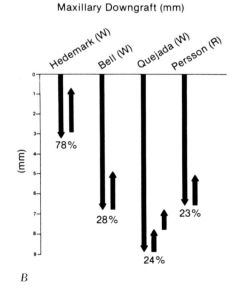

B

FIGURE 10–12   Tabular (*A*) and graphic (*B*) representations of the changes during and after maxillary downgrafts.

postoperative) suggest some improvement but still leave many questions unanswered. Hedemark's[46] 78 percent relapse figure is reflective of the findings of many early researchers who saw considerable superior relapse following maxillary downgrafts. Once bone grafting and auxiliary fixation procedures such as Steinmann pins[20] were introduced, relapse rates with wire fixation (i.e., Bell 28 percent)[47] were considerably reduced. More recently, the addition of rigid fixation and hydroxylapatite interpositional grafts offers the potential for improved stability, although this has not been clearly demonstrated in the available literature to this date.[48,49]

SUMMARY

The past decade has seen a considerable improvement in long-term stability following mandibular advancement as the transition from interdental to skeletal wiring for postsurgical fixation occurred. The introduction of rigid fixation, while having halved the incidence of relapse, has offered only a moderate improvement over current skeletal fixation techniques in those cases showing postsurgical instability. Of prime importance to the clinician is the fact that mandibular advancement cases with rigid fixation that undergo relapse frequently do so in an anterior direction rather than in the posterior direction usually seen with wire fixation. Care should therefore be taken with the long-term use of Class II elastics in rigid fixation cases if a high relapse potential is suspected.

Although it has received less publicity than mandibular advancements, the relapse of mandibular setbacks with wire fixation appears to be similar both in incidence and amount. Larger setbacks in particular seem to be prone to greater relapse, and as yet there are insufficient data on the effects of rigid fixation to tell if it will have a significant effect. The initial findings of different relapse patterns between sagittal splits and transoral vertical ramus osteotomies need further investigation because they have considerable clinical implications, particularly in cases in which future mandibular growth is a possibility.

Isolated maxillary impaction with wire fixation appears from the data to be a more stable procedure than mandibular advancement, with only 20 percent of the cases showing significant relapse compared to 40 percent for the mandibular surgeries. In addition, the amount of change, often around only 1 mm, was considerably less than that seen in the mandible. Proffit's data seem to suggest that segmenting the maxilla has no effect on vertical stability. However, more evaluation of changes in the transverse and anteroposterior planes, as well as comparison of two- and three-segment surgeries, is required before a definite conclusion can be reached on this point.

When maxillary impaction is carried out in conjunction with mandibular advancement there appears to be no deterioration in maxillary vertical stability. In fact, in this case rigid fixation appears to improve stability, primarily by reducing the clockwise rotation of the jaws frequently seen after two jaw surgery with wire fixation. Rigid fixation also improves maxillary vertical stability by virtually eliminating large relapses (i.e., those greater than 2 mm). The findings for the mandibular advancement component of the double jaw cases were similar, with equal or slightly improved stability being noted for both the wire and particularly the rigid fixation samples.

The long-term data for both maxillary advancements and maxillary downgrafts suggest that with contemporary techniques one can expect relapse of about 20 percent in the posterior and superior directions, respectively. The effects of rigid fixation and various interpositional grafting techniques remain inconclusive at this time. As with all the other procedures, considerably more long-term data, preferably up to five years postsurgery, are required before an adequate picture of the long-term stability of orthognathic surgery can be painted.

REFERENCES

1. Poulton DR, Ware WH: Surgical-orthodontic treatment of severe mandibular retrusion: Part I. Am J Orthod 59:244–265, 1971.
2. Poulton DR, Ware WH: Surgical-orthodontic treatment of severe mandibular retrusion: Part II. Am J Orthod 63:237–255, 1973.
3. Wilmar K: On LeFort I osteotomy: A follow-up study of 106 operated patients with maxillofacial deformity. Scan J Plast Reconstr Surg Supp 12:1–68, 1974.
4. McNeill RW, Hooley JR, Sundberg RJ: Skeletal relapse during intermaxillary fixation. J Oral Surg 31:212–227, 1973.
5. Ive J, McNeill RW, West RA: Mandibular advancement: Skeletal and dental changes during fixation. J Oral Surg 37:881–886, 1977.
6. Kohn MW: Analysis of relapse after mandibular advancement surgery. J Oral Surg 36:676–684, 1978.
7. Schendel SA, Epker BN: Results after mandibular advancement surgery: An analysis of 87 cases. J Oral Surg 38:265–282, 1980.
8. Lake SL, McNeill RW, Little RM, West RA: Surgical mandibular advancement: A cephalometric analysis of treatment response. Am J Orthod 80:376–394, 1981.
9. Schendel SA, Eisenfeld JH, Bell WH, Epker BN: Superior repositioning of the maxilla: Stability and soft tissue osseous relations. Am J Orthod 70:663–674, 1976.
10. Hedemark A, Freihofer HP Jr: The behavior of the maxilla in vertical movements after LeFort I osteotomy. J Maxillofacial Surg 6:244–249, 1978.
11. Brammer J, Finn R, Bell WH, Sinn D, Reisch J, Dana K: Stability after bimaxillary surgery to correct vertical maxillary excess and mandibular deficiency. J Oral Surg 38:664–670, 1980.
12. McNamara JA, Carlson DS, Yellich GM, Hendricksen RP: Musculoskeletal adaptation following orthognathic surgery. *In* Carlson DS, McNamara JA (eds.): Muscle Adaptation in the Craniofacial Region. Monograph No. 8, Craniofacial Growth Series. Ann Arbor, MI, Center for Human Growth and Development, University of Michigan, 1978, pp. 91–132.

13. Epker BN, Wolford LM, Fish LC: Mandibular deficiency syndrome: II. Surgical considerations for mandibular advancement. Oral Surg 45:349–363, 1978.
14. Worms FW, Speidel TM, Bevis RR, Waite DE: Posttreatment stability esthetics of orthognathic surgery. Angle Orthod 50:251–273, 1980.
15. Epker BN, Wessberg GA: Mechanisms of early skeletal relapse following surgical advancement of the mandible. Br J Oral Surg 20:175–182, 1982.
16. Reitzik M: Mandibular advancement surgery: Stability following a modified fixation technique. J Oral Surg 31:516–521, 1973.
17. Steinhauser EW: Advancement of the mandible by sagittal ramus split and suprahyoid myotomy: An experimental study. J Oral Surg 31:516–521, 1973.
18. Ellis E III, Carlson DS: Stability two years after mandibular advancement with and without suprahyoid myotomy: An experimental study. J Oral Maxillofacial Surg 41:426–437, 1983.
19. Booth DF: Control of the proximal fragment by lower border wiring in the sagittal split osteotomy. J Maxillofacial Surg 9:126–128, 1981.
20. Bennett MA, Wolford LM: The maxillary step osteotomy and Steinmann pin stabilization. J Oral Maxillofacial Surg 43:307–311, 1985.
21. Champy M, Lodde JP, Schmitt R, Jaeger JH, Muster D: Mandibular osteosynthesis by miniature screwed plates via a buccal approach. J Maxillofacial Surg 6:14–21, 1978.
22. Ellis E, Gallow WJ: Relapse following mandibular advancement with dental plus skeletal fixation. J Oral Maxillofacial Surg 44:509–513, 1986.
23. Thomas PM, Tucker MR, Prewitt JR, Proffit WR: Early skeletal and dental changes following mandibular advancement and rigid internal fixation. Int J Adult Orthod Orthog Surg 1:171–178, 1986.
24. Luyk NH, Ward-Booth RP: The stability of LeFort I advancement osteotomies using bone plates without bone grafts. J Maxillofacial Surg 13:250–253, 1985.
25. Sandor GK, Stoelinga RJ, Tideman H: The role of intraosseous osteosynthesis wire in sagittal split osteotomies for mandibular advancement. J Oral Maxillofacial Surg 32:231, 1984.
26. Watske IM, Turvey TA, Phillips C, Proffit WR: Stability of mandibular after sagittal osteotomy with screw or wire fixation: A comparative study. J Oral Maxillofacial Surg 48:108–121, 1990.
27. Simmons KE, Phillips C, Turvey TA: Five year follow-up of surgical orthodontic mandibular deficiency by sagittal osteotomy. Int J Adult Orthod Orthog Surg 7:67–79, 1992.
28. Caskey RT, Turpin DL, Bloomquist D: Stability of mandibular lengthening using bicortical screw fixation. Am J Orthod 96:320–326, 1989.
29. Barrer PG, Wallen TR, McNeill RW, Reitzik M: Stability of mandibular advancement osteotomy using rigid internal fixation. Am J Orthod 92:403–411, 1987.
30. Van Sickels JE, Larsen AJ, Thrash WJ: Relapse after rigid fixation of mandibular advancement. J Oral Maxillofacial Surg 44:698–702, 1986.
31. Kobayashi T, Watanabe I, Uede K: Stability of the mandible after sagittal ramus osteotomy for the correction of prognathism. J Oral Maxillofacial Surg 44:693–697, 1986.
32. Rosenquist B, Rune B, Selvik G: Displacement of the mandible after removal of the intermaxillary fixation following oblique sliding osteotomy. J Oral Maxillofacial Surg 14:251–259, 1986.

33. Astrand P, Ridell A: Positional changes of the mandible and the upper and lower teeth after oblique sliding osteotomy of the mandibular rami. Scand J Plast Reconstr Surg 7:120, 1973.

34. Vijayaraghavan K, Richardson A, Witlock R: Postoperative relapse following sagittal split osteotomy. Br J Oral Surg 12:63, 1974.

35. Phillips C, Zaytoun HS, Thomas PM, Terry BC: Skeletal alterations following TOVRO or BSSO procedures. Int J Adult Ortho Orthog Surg 3:203–213, 1986.

36. Franco JE, Van Sickels JE Thrash WJ: Factors contributing to relapse in rigidly fixed mandibular setbacks. J Oral Maxillofacial Surg 47:451–456, 1989.

37. Greebe RB, Tuinzing DB: Superior repositioning of the maxilla by a LeFort I osteotomy. Oral Surg Oral Med Oral Pathol 63:158–161, 1987.

38. Proffit WR, Phillips C, Turvey TA: Stability following superior repositioning of the maxilla by LeFort I osteotomy. Am J Orthod Dentofacial Orthop 92:151–161, 1987.

39. Bishara SE, Chu GW, Jakobsen J: Stability of the LeFort I one-piece maxillary osteotomy. Am J Orthod Dentofacial Orthop 94:184–200, 1988.

40. Turvey TA, Phillips C, Zaytoun HS, Proffit WR: Simultaneous superior repositioning of the maxilla and mandibular advancement. Am J Orthod Dentofacial Orthop 94:372–382, 1988.

41. Satrom KD, Sinclair PM, Wolford LM: The stability of double jaw surgery: A comparison of rigid versus wire fixation. Am J Orthod Dentofacial Orthop 99:550–563, 1991.

42. Hennes JA, Wallen RT, Bloomquist DS, Crouch DL: Stability of simultaneous mobilization of the maxilla and mandible utilizing internal rigid fixation. Int J Adult Orthod Orthog Surg 3:127–141, 1988.

43. Teuscher U, Sailer HF: The stability of LeFort I osteotomy in Class III cases with retropositioned maxillae. J Maxillofacial Surg 10:80–83, 1982.

44. Weiss MJ, Patty S, Phillips C: Dental and skeletal stability following maxillary advancement. J Dent Res 68:259 (abstr. 625), 1989.

45. Wardrop RW, Wolford LM: Maxillary stability following downgraft and/or advancement procedures with stabilization using rigid fixation and poray block hydroxylapatite implants. J Oral Maxillofacial Surg 47:336–342, 1989.

46. Hedemark A, Freihofer HP: The behavior of the maxilla in vertical movements after the LeFort I osteotomy. J Oral Maxillofacial Surg 6:244, 1978.

47. Bell WH, Scheideman GB: Correction of vertical maxillary deficiency: Stability and soft tissue changes. J Oral Maxillofacial Surg 39:666–670, 1981.

48. Quejada H, Bell W, Kawamura H, Zhang X: Skeletal stability after inferior maxillary positioning. Int J Adult Orthod Orthog Surg 2:67–74, 1987.

49. Persson G, Hellem S, Nord PG: Bone plates for stabilizing LeFort I osteotomies. J Oral Maxillofacial Surg 14:69–73, 1986.

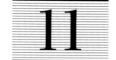
Biomechanical Aspects of Stability of Occlusion

Dietmar Kubein-Meesenburg
and Hans Nägerl

INTRODUCTION

One of the most important unsolved problems in orthodontics is the long-term stability of the treatment's result. Are relapses a consequence only of insufficient treatment, or can permanent stability be lost as a result of natural variations? The stomatognathic system, and especially the occlusion, is in a steady state, like the entire body. This state presumably is unstable as variations such as horizontal and vertical abrasion, which are programmed into the stomatognathic system and which are responsible for stabilizing the teeth, no longer occur given our style of life.

On the other hand, an ideal picture of static alignment and arrangement of the occlusal surfaces and elements (teeth and TMJs) can be established biomechanically and statistically supported. In centric occlusion, for example, the TMJs are biomechanically positioned in centric relation at the transition from the fossa to the protuberantia. One consequence of this ideal static arrangement is the optimal mechanical functioning of the kinematics and dynamics of the mandible's cranial border movement. In physics, this border movement constitutes that of a couple in a special force-locked gear system that operates in protrusion as well as in retrusion. The centric occlusion is characterized by the switching of the mandible from the protrusive to the retrusive gear system, and vice versa. The individual biomechanical mechanism can be described for the entire occlusion and may be compared with the empirically and experimentally

171

proved ideal mechanism. If these biomechanical laws are taken into account in diagnosis and therapy, results may be achieved in orthodontics that stand up over the long term.

In the following section, the basic biomechanics of the occlusal elements are decribed in order to point out the special significance of centric occlusion for kinematic and dynamic stability. Special attention is given to the biomechanical significance of the curve of Spee, since it demonstrates the hierarchical structure of the stomatognathic system. Through this an essential is structurally given for the long-term stability of the steady state of occlusion.

IDEAL BIOMECHANICAL ARRANGEMENT OF OCCLUSAL ELEMENTS

POSTERIOR OCCLUSAL ELEMENTS

FUNCTION OF THE TMJ.   The biomechanical mechanism of the TMJs can be understood through an examination of TMJ morphology. It can be verified through radiological, or even better, through axiographic measurements. At first, the articular disc of the TMJ may be neglected in the biomechanical analysis because its significance is relatively small in the structure of the cranial border movement. In pure protrusion, the condyle slides along a sigmoid curve almost without friction (Fig. 11–1). This frictionless movement determines that at rest the condyle (mandible) can load only the os temporale (maxilla) with forces whose resultant F (force) is perpendicular to the two articular surfaces. Therefore, in a sagittal plane, the force line must be vertical to the two contours of the condyle and the os temporale. The tangents in the loading points of the contours are parallel (Fig. 11–2). At a point of inflection, the inclination of the corresponding tangent is at an extreme. This means that if the application line of the resultant F intersects the inflection point of the sigmoid contour of the os temporale, the articular contour (surface) of the

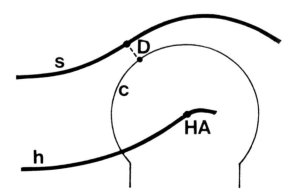

FIGURE 11–1   Function of TMJ. s = sagittal contour of the maxillary guiding surface; c = sagittal contour of the condyle; D = minimum thickness of the intermediar zone of the disc; h = path of hinge axis; HA = hinge axis in CR. c slides along s.

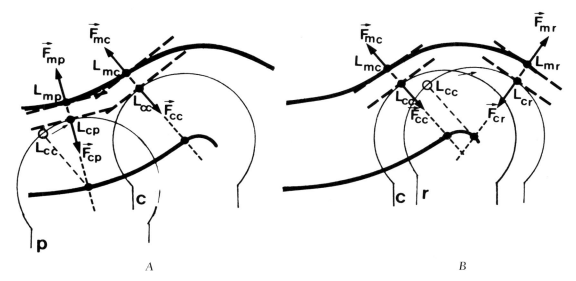

A   *B*

FIGURE 11–2   Loading points. The tangents (dashed lines) through corresponding loading points (L_{mp}/L_{cp}, L_{mc}/L_{cc}, L_{mr}/L_{cr}) are parallel. The position of the condyle (c) = centric relation. The resultant forces F_{mp}, F_{mc}, and F_{mr} onto the maxillary guiding surfaces have the opposite sign of the corresponding loads of the condyle.
A, Protrusion. Though the condyle moves forward, the loading point migrates retrusively ($L_{cc} \rightarrow L_{cp}$). B, Retrusion. When the condyle moves a little bit backward, the loading point retrusively migrates over the entire articular surface of the condyle ($L_{cc}, \rightarrow L_{cr}$). In both cases the force vectors possess the same direction of rotation. Only their rotational centers are different.

condyle will be met by this line at the most anterior point (Fig. 11–2). This relation of the most anterior loading point on the condyle to the inflection point of the os temporale constitutes the centric relation of the TMJ. Ideally, this position coincides with centric occlusion.

This coincidence yields the following pattern of movement of the loading points: In protrusion, as well as in retrusion, the loading point on the condyle migrates backward on the contour. In the left condylus, this point runs clockwise on the almost circular contour. The corresponding loading point migrates forward on the eminentia and backward on the fossa. In both cases the resultant force vector rotates clockwise (Fig. 11–2). A more retruded relation of the condyle to the os temporale, coinciding with centric occlusion, means a reduction of the mandible's retrusive space of movement and a change in the direction of rotation of the resultant force vector in the joint during protrusion. Undoubtedly, the change in the direction of rotation should induce problems of control for the related musculature. An anterior position of centric relation in combination with centric occlusion results in a reduction of the protrusive articular surface on the condyle and in the same problems as in the mandible, as just described. In addition, the coincidence of centric relation and centric occlusion can be confirmed by further arguments and findings:

1. The thickness of the cartilage and the density of the bone at their maximum at the inflection area of the os temporale. This coincides with the fact that the joint is most frequently and most strongly loaded when the mandible is in centric occlusion.

2. In protusion, the articular disc slides together with the condyle so that the minimum thickness of the disc (intermediate zone) lies between the two loading points (on the condyle and on the eminentia) along the entire protrusive path. If, however, the disc is guided together with the condyle out of a protruded position backward, the relation "minimum thickness between the two loading points" will be fulfilled only up to the inflection point. If the inflection point is surpassed, the condyle will run onto the motionless posterior band of the disc.[1] In addition, the centric relation of the joint separates two different functions of the disc.

3. Analysis of the relation of the measurements of the bony surfaces of macerated skulls (with almost complete dentition, Angle Class I relation) indicated that 39 of 40 skulls possessed the ideal arrangement: centric relation = centric occlusion.[2]

POSTERIOR CRANIAL GUIDANCE IN PROTRUSION AND RETRUSION

In centric relation the disc takes its most distocranial position, in which it can become deposited with minimum thickness (of the intermediate zone) between the os temporale and the condyle. When the condyle glides along its cranial border anteriorly (that is, with minimum distance along the os temporale), the path of the hinge axis is a magnified picture of the sagittal contour of the protuberantia articularis. In first approximation this path is circular. The hinge axis moves around a fixed, maxillary rotational axis (Fig. 11–3). In pure protrusion the function of the joint can be reduced to a dimeric chain (Fig. 11–3B). The distance between both axes, the rod of the chain, is given by the sum of the radii of curvature of the eminentia and the condyle plus the minimum thickness of the disc.[3]

In retrusion, the condyle runs onto the posterior band of the disk and the ligamentary limitation. The resulting measurable path of the hinge axis depends upon the shape and volume of the fossa and the condyle and upon the cartilaginous and fibrous structures (posterior band, ligamentary limitation, and so on). In a first approximation this retrusive path also represents a circle. The retrusive function of the joint can also be reduced to a dimeric chain (Fig. 11–4). The circle of curvature of the hinge axis path again is the distance between the fixed maxillary axis and the fixed mandibular (hinge) axis.[3] The position of centric relation of the

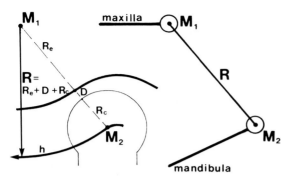

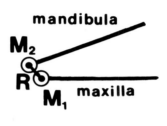

FIGURE 11–3 Protrusive function of the TMJ.

A, The hinge axis (M_2) runs out of centric relation along an almost circular path (h) with the center of curvature (M_1). The distance (R) between M_2 and M_1 is practically constant. The TMJ possesses *two* rotational axes, M_2 and M_1. *B*, The principal functioning of the TMJ in protrusion as a kinematically open, dimeric link chain. The length of the rod (R) equals the radius (R_e) of the eminence, the minimum thickness (D) of the intermediary zone of the disc, and the radius (R_c) of the condyle.

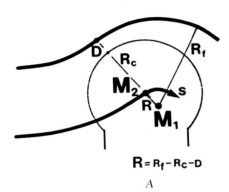

$$R = R_f - R_c - D$$

A

B

FIGURE 11–4 Retrusive function of the TMJ.

A, The hinge axis (M_2) runs out of centric relation along an almost circular path (s) with the center of curvature (M_1). The distance (R) between M_2 and M_1 is practically constant. The TMJ possesses *two* rotational axes, M_2 and M_1. In comparison with the protrusive function, the centers M_2 and M_1 have changed places and lie close together. *B*, The principal functioning of the TMJ in retrusion as a kinematically open, dimeric link chain. Considering the direction of the path of the hinge axis, the maxillary center (M_1) lies at the right side, just as in protrusion.

condyle is given by the gap of curvature on the axiographic tracing at the anterior end of its retrusive cute tail. This position ideally and regularly coincides with centric occlusion.[1,2]

ARTICULAR SPACE OF MOVEMENT

In the retrusive function, the condyle slides onto the posterior band. The same relative motion occurs at any protruded position of the condyle when the disc is drawn forward by the the caput superior of the m. pterygoideus lat. Schumacher[4] wrote:

> The effective force line of the caput superior is not identical to the direction

of the muscular tract, since the muscle is inserted in the disk and thus gets hypomochlion from the tuberculum articulare. Because of this arrangement of angles the horizontal action is transformed into a lowering movement of the mandible.

Thus, the condyle has a component of movement that is vertical to the guiding structure of the os temporale. It gains a clearance, and the mandible can—guided by the muscular apparatus—float in space. The occlusal element that is most posteriorly positioned, the TMJ, possesses not only a cranial border guidance but also an articular movement space. Structurally this space corresponds to the Posselt diagram, which defines the movement space of the lower incisal edge. This machinery makes it possible for the mandible to function during chewing as a free lever arm whose pivot bearing is positioned at the hypomochlion (as Motsch[5] has already described). Only by this means can the entire force of the muscular apparatus be applied onto the bolus. Consequently, the TMJs then are free of load.

ANTERIOR OCCLUSAL ELEMENTS

STATICS OF INCISAL ARRANGEMENTS

Anterior guidance is given by the palatal surfaces of the maxillary incisors. The lower incisal edges glide almost without friction along the palatal vault. In pure protrusion, the path of an incisal edge is given by the sagittal contour of the guiding surface. A force can be applied from one tooth onto another only when the vector is perpendicular to the common tangent of both teeth (Fig. 11–5). Therefore, the two touching incisal teeth represent a joint whose ideal centric relation is given by the relation of a lower incisor to the inflection point (B_p) from the palatal concavity to convexity; only in this relation are the torques that twist the incisal skeletal bases minimal (Fig. 11–5A). Any other relation yields an increase of torque load, especially onto the mandibular incisor. This ideal centric relation coincides biomechanically with the centric occlusion of the mandible.[1] Since the mandible can rotate around the hinge axis (with a small angle) without altering its centric relation, the longitudinal axis of the mandibular incisor should ideally coincide with a tangent of a circle around the hinge axis.[1,6,7] This means that in CO/CR relation of the incisal joint the tangent in B_p has to meet the hinge axis (Fig. 11–6). This arrangement is the most frequent one, even in new orthodontic cases.[1]

STRUCTURE OF THE ANTERIOR PROTRUSIVE GUIDANCE

It can be shown that all sagittal contour curves of the palatal concavity have the same shape (within accuracy of measurement) and that all con-

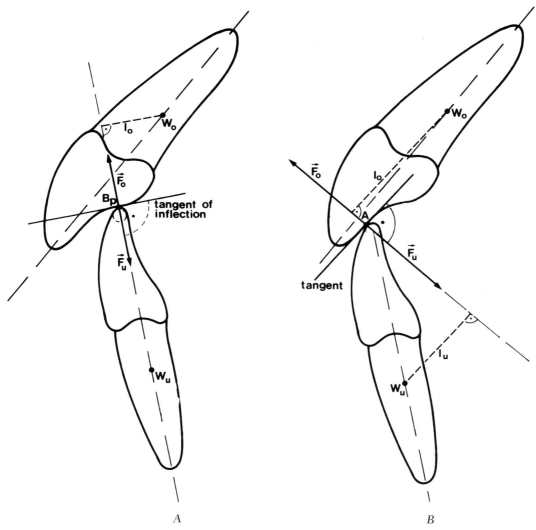

FIGURE 11–5 In the incisal joint (the contact point must be regarded as a joint), both incisors are stressed by forces whose vectors are perpendicular to the joint's tangents.

A, The ideal centric relation of the incisal joint (IT). When the lower incisal edge meets the base point (B_p) and the long axis is perpendicular to the tangent in B_p, the torsional stress of the skeletal bases of the two teeth possesses its minimum value. *B,* Protruded relation of the incisal joint (IT). The skeletal basis of the lower incisor is especially stressed by an increased torque.

tour curves of one individual can be approximated by the same catenary.[8,9] Therefore, all these curves posses the same initial radius of curvature. In pure protrusion, the incisor joint can also structurally be reduced to a dimeric chain (Fig. 11–7).[3]

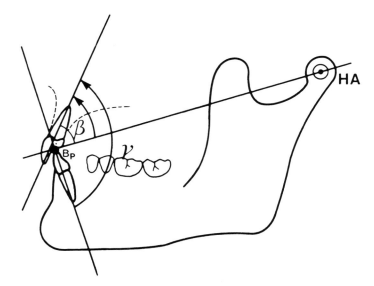

FIGURE 11–6   Ideal statisics of the incisal joint. The tangent in the inflection point (B_p) passes the hinge axis (HA). The long axis of the lower incisor is perpendicular to this tangent. The interincisal angle $\alpha = \beta - 90°$. β = an individual morphological angle.

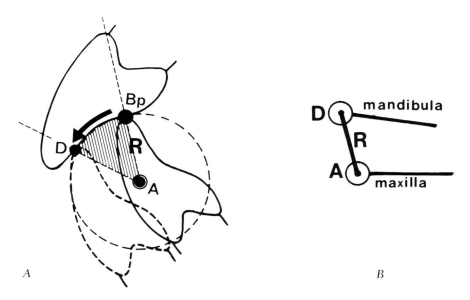

FIGURE 11–7   The principal functioning of the incisal joint.
A, In protrusion, starting from the base point (B_p), the mandibular incisal edge (D) runs along an almost circular path with the fixed maxillary center (A). The incisal joint consists of *two* rotational axes (D and A), which hold the constant distance (R). *B*, The principal functioning of the protrusive incisal joint as a kinematically open, dimeric chain.

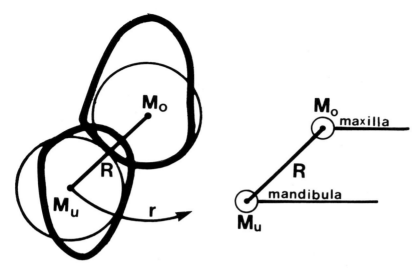

FIGURE 11–8   The principal functioning of the premolar joint.
A, In retrusion, the lower premolar slides along the upper one. In first approximation the two contours can be replaced by their circles of curvature. The center
(M_u) runs along the retrusive circular path (r) around M_o. The premolar joint
consists of *two* rotational axes (M_o and M_u) in the distance R. *B*, The principal
functioning of the retrusive premolar joint as a kinematically open, dimeric
chain.

STRUCTURE OF THE ANTERIOR RETRUSIVE GUIDANCE

Since the incisors disclude when the mandible retrusively moves out of
centric occlusion, the dominant anterior guidance is adopted by the most
anteriorly positioned retrusive guiding facets (usually the first premolars).
The other teeth disclude. The two sliding contours of these premolars also
represent a dimeric chain (Fig. 11–8).

BIOMECHANICAL LINKAGE BETWEEN ANTERIOR AND POSTERIOR GUIDANCE

PROTRUSION

From centric occlusion, the mandible can execute a purely protrusive
plane movement in the sagittal-vertical planes. When the mandible (of
Class I patients) glides along its cranial border, the (potential) protrusive
guidances of the molar region are separated because of the dominance of
the most anterior and most posterior guidances represented by the
incisors and the TMJ. As in physics, this cranial border movement (determined by the rigid linkage between anterior and posterior guidance) con-

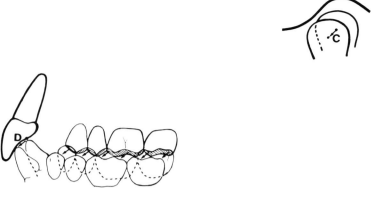

FIGURE 11–9   Protrusive cranial border movement. The mandible is guided by the incisal joint and the TMJ. The other teeth disclude. The mandible moves with positive drive. This mechanism is called the cam gear.

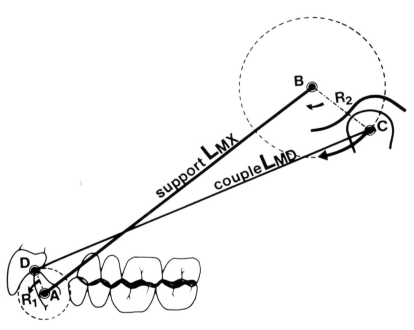

FIGURE 11–10   The protrusive link quadrangle of the stomatognathic system. The movable couple (DC) rotates with its two ends around the fixed maxillary centers (A and B). DC = couple = functional length of the mandible, L_{MD}; AB = support = functional length of the maxilla, L_{MX}.

stitutes the movement of a couple in a force-locked cam gear (Fig. 11–9). Since the anterior as well as the posterior function of articulation (in its initial phase) can be replaced by dimeric chains in the abstract, the stomatognathic gear system can be modeled by a link quadrangle (Fig. 11–10). This stomatognathic link quadrangle has special properties in physics.[10,11]

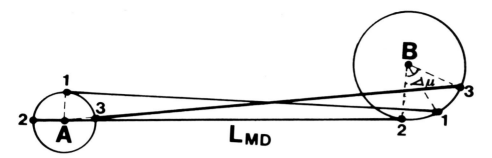

FIGURE 11–11 Definition of the posterior oscillating angle ($\Delta\mu$). (1) Initial position of the mandible; (2) anterior dead position; (3) posterior dead position.

Technologically, it constitutes a throttle crank whose anterior (smaller) wheel can rotate 360°, whereas the posterior wheel only oscillates. The sides of this corresponding oscillating angle, $\Delta\mu$, are related to the anterior and posterior dead positions of the gear system (Fig. 11–11). The oscillating angle, $\Delta\mu$, is an interindividual human constant, like blood pressure or body temperature. Its average value is $\Delta\mu = 23°$.[10,11]

In order to describe the kinematic state of the system, the so-called fixed centrode (holoide), which represents the geometrical loci of the momentary rotational centers of the mandible, is used. From its incipient position P_{prot}—the protrusive rotational center of the mandible in centric occlusion—this center migrates cranially to infinity and returns caudally (Fig. 11–12). For Class I cases this fixed centrode closely conforms to its asymptote, so that the curved and straight lines practically coincide. Only this very special part is physiologically used. This special property not only possesses the approximate model link quadrangle, but more precisely it is kept by the complete, existing individual cam gear.[12]

Result: The protrusive fixed centrode can be replaced by its asymptote within the complete functional range of the palatally guided protrusive gear system.

This quasilinearity of the functional range of the fixed centrode has a profound mechanical significance: A resultant force vector of the muscles that acts along this line produces a neutral equilibrium of the mandible. The mandible can be moved without being influenced by this force. In addition, the asymptote practically constitutes the borderline between the mechanically stable and unstable equilibria of the mandible (Fig. 11–13).

RETRUSION

From centric occlusion the mandible can also move distally.[1,2] Analogous to the protrusion for this movement, the dominant guidance is given by the most anterior and most posterior guiding facets (the first premolars

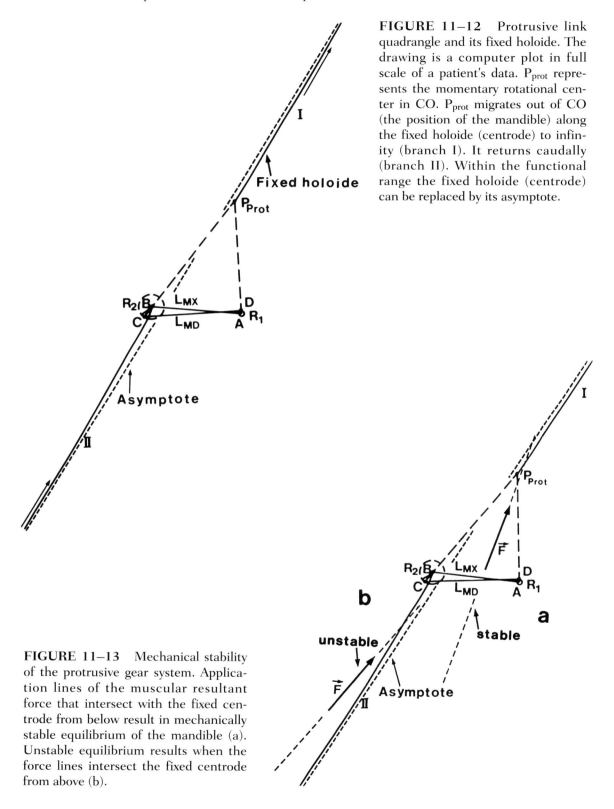

FIGURE 11–12 Protrusive link quadrangle and its fixed holoide. The drawing is a computer plot in full scale of a patient's data. P_{prot} represents the momentary rotational center in CO. P_{prot} migrates out of CO (the position of the mandible) along the fixed holoide (centrode) to infinity (branch I). It returns caudally (branch II). Within the functional range the fixed holoide (centrode) can be replaced by its asymptote.

FIGURE 11–13 Mechanical stability of the protrusive gear system. Application lines of the muscular resultant force that intersect with the fixed centrode from below result in mechanically stable equilibrium of the mandible (a). Unstable equilibrium results when the force lines intersect the fixed centrode from above (b).

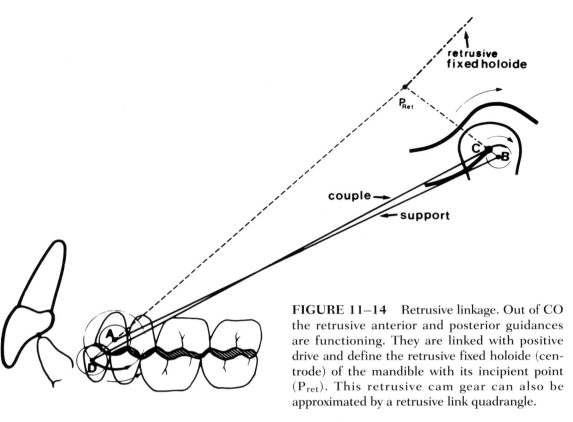

FIGURE 11–14 Retrusive linkage. Out of CO the retrusive anterior and posterior guidances are functioning. They are linked with positive drive and define the retrusive fixed holoide (centrode) of the mandible with its incipient point (P_{ret}). This retrusive cam gear can also be approximated by a retrusive link quadrangle.

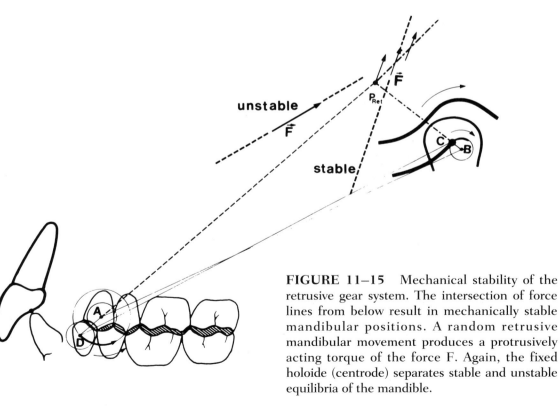

FIGURE 11–15 Mechanical stability of the retrusive gear system. The intersection of force lines from below result in mechanically stable mandibular positions. A random retrusive mandibular movement produces a protrusively acting torque of the force F. Again, the fixed holoide (centrode) separates stable and unstable equilibria of the mandible.

and the TMJ, respectively). The potentially retrusive facets in between disclude. This retrusive mandibular function also operates like a cam gear in physics. Since anterior and posterior articulation can be reduced to dimeric chains, the cam gear also represents a link quadrangle. The corresponding fixed centrode (holoide) runs distally/cranially starting from the initial momentary rotational center P_{ret} given by centric occlusion (Fig. 11–14). This curve again separates stable and unstable mandibular equilibria. Force lines of the muscles that intersect this line from below produce stable states. A steep, retrusive fixed centrode increases the probability of mechanical instability (Fig. 11–15).

THE SWITCHING MECHANISM BETWEEN THE PROTRUSIVE AND RETRUSIVE MANDIBULAR GEAR SYSTEM

THEORY AND FINDINGS

The transition from the protrusive to the retrusive mandibular function is of special interest from a biomechanical view. This transition is defined by centric occlusion and is related to the centric relation of the TMJ. In this position, the cranial movements of the mandible are determined by two different momentary rotational centers: P_{prot} and P_{ret} (Fig. 11–16). Since the posterior guidance uses the same guiding surfaces for both types of movements, both initial rotational centers lie on the same posterior radial vector. In the retrusive direction, the retrusive system operates by switching the anterior guidance from the incisors to the premolars, and vice versa for the protrusive direction. The transition from protrusion to retrusion is characterized by a jump from the protrusive to the retrusive fixed centrode and vice versa for retrusion to protrusion (Fig. 11–16).

The discontinuity of the fixed centrode at centric occlusion and its interaction with the resultant force of the muscular apparatus give a high degree of mechanical stability to this mandibular position. The cranial border movement and, therefore, the two series-connected gear systems, function only on the condition that the sliding surfaces are force locked. Muscular forces, which may be small, have to press the mandible by means of the related ligaments onto its defined maxillary cranial border in order to produce the corresponding guiding contracts. According to the position of the resultant force line, the mandible occupies protruded or retruded positions or the particularly stable position of centric occlusion (Fig. 11–17). All force vectors whose lines run between the initial centers P_{prot} and P_{ret} and do not meet one of the fixed centrodes hold the mandible mechanically stable in centric occlusion. In order to reach centric occlusion, the muscular apparatus has only to produce a force vector lying between the two centers P_{prot} and P_{ret}. *An exact adjustment of the force vector is not necessary.* The centric occlusion defines a certain *region of stability* for the acting muscular apparatus. In contrast, any other position of the mandible at the cranial border is produced by only one resultant force line that lies outside this occlusal region of stability.

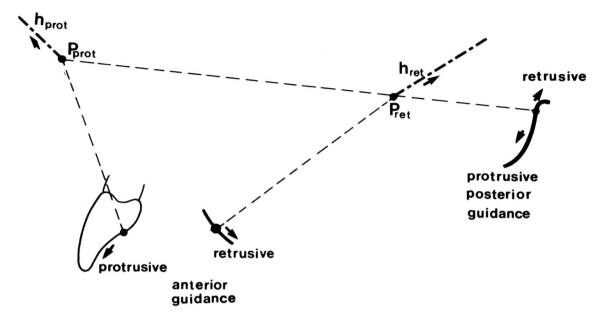

FIGURE 11–16 Kinematic significance of the CO/CR position of the mandible. In CO/CR the mandible has two momentary centers of rotation that operate according to the direction of movement. This splitting is produced by the anterior guidance that jumps from the protrusive incisal guidance to the retrusive premolar guidance. The two centers (P_{prot} and P_{ret}) are the origins of the protrusive and retrusive fixed centrodes (h_{prot} and h_{ret}, respectively).

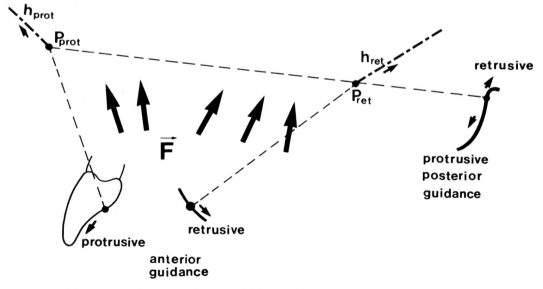

FIGURE 11–17 Stability of the mandible in CO/CR. Every resultant force vector (F) of the muscles that lie between the two rotational centers (P_{prot} and P_{ret}) that does not meet one of the fixed centrodes (holoides) holds the mandible in CO/CR position.

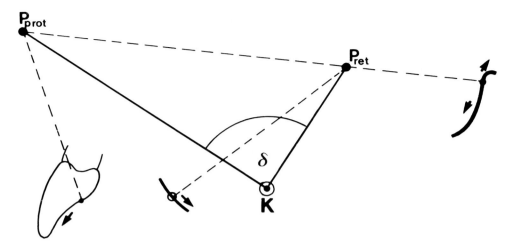

FIGURE 11–18   Definition of angle of stability (δ). K = center of mastication.

In order to describe the range of stability quantitatively, the angle of stability (δ) was determined to be defined by the two initial centers P_{prot} and P_{ret} and the center of mastication as angle vertex (Fig. 11–18). The center of mastication was assumed to be at the first molars. The measurements were taken from 39 macerated skulls with Angle Class I relation. The skulls were fixed in centric occlusion and analyzed by lateral X-rays (for details of measuring equipment and methods, see reference 2). All skulls showed the biomechanically ideal, unequivocal relation of the condyles to the transition from the fossa to the tuberculum articulare and with that the coincidence of centric occlusion with centric relation. In the incisor region, the biomechanically ideal relation of the lower incisal edge to the basepoint B_p of the palatal concavity was found only in 50 percent (20) of the skulls. The other 19 skulls possessed an anteposition of the incisal contact point up to a maximum of 6 mm (average value 3.7 mm) measured from the basepoint. To re-emphasize the point, this anteposition does not influence the ideal centric relation of the TMJ. Table 11–1 shows the simple statistics of the angle δ for ideal and nonideal incisor relation. The two samples are scarcely statistically differentiated. The t-test of the

TABLE 11–1   Simple Statistics of the Angle of Stability (δ)

	Incisor Relation	
	Ideal	*Protruded*
Average	55,15°	61,1°
Standard deviation	15,5°	13,4°
Maximum value	77°	80°
Minimum value	32°	32°

difference of average $\Delta\delta = 5.8°$ results in a probability of the zero hypothesis being more than 10 percent. Both variances are homogeneous (F-test).

Result: The region of stability seen from the center of mastication is spread over a relatively large angle that is scarcely influenced by the biomechanical relation of the incisors. At most, one can suppose a trend, with deviations from the biomechanical ideal being accompanied by an increase of the region of stability.

THE SWITCHING MECHANISM

In CO/CR the anterior guidance switches from the protrusive to the retrusive function, and vice versa. The guide rail jumps from the incisors onto the premolars. Exactly at centric occlusion the path of a lower incisal edge has a discontinuity of its gradient and, therefore, of its differential coefficient of the first order. These findings are independent of the position of the incisal contact, whether it is ideal (at B_p) or anterior to B_p.

At centric relation the path of the hinge axis also shows a special feature. The curvature changes its sign. The center of the circle of curvature jumps from one side of the path to the other side. It is logically consistent that this rapid variation of the differential coefficient of the second order in the posterior guidance coincides with the discontinuity of the anterior guidance. This is further proof of the biomechanical significance of the relation between centric relation and centric occlusion as coincident mandibular positions.

For this switching mechanism of the combined protrusive and retrusive gear system, the biomechanically ideal static arrangement of the incisors is not necessary: The tangent of inflection in B_p does not need to run through the hinge axis, the incisors' contact point does not have to be at B_p, and the lower incisal long axis does not need to be a tangent of a circle around the hinge axis. At first only the minimizing of the stress of the incisal skeletal bases brings about this ideal arrangement of the incisors. Other hierarchical factors can require a deviation from this ideal static arrangement of the incisors. On the other hand, the anteposition of the incisor contact (compared to the ideal contact point B_p) often has the advantage of a wider region of stability.

Stability in centric occlusion is not completely described by the angle of stability alone. Force lines through the center of mastication that lie within the angle of stability can cut the retrusive fixed centrode from above when its slope is too steep (Fig. 11–19). Such a case would produce a mechanically unstable equilibrium of the mandible. For the muscular apparatus to hold the corresponding position of the mandible, it would have to balance. Control oscillations would occur. Such an instability can arise when the radius of curvature of the retrusive path of the hinge axis is too long, as seen in TMJ cases.

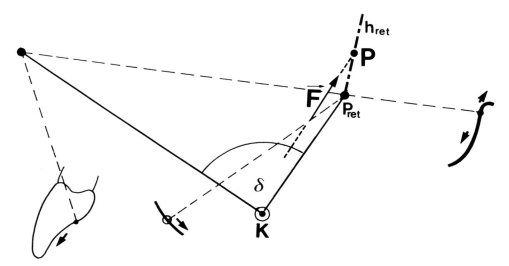

FIGURE 11–19   Retrusive instability. Although the force (F) lies within the region of stability, it produces an unstable, retrusive mandibular position (P). This happens when the retrusive fixed centrode is positioned too steeply (drawing not in full scale).

ALIGNMENT OF THE PROTRUSIVE GEAR SYSTEM IN THE SKULL

Theory and empiricism[11,12] of the protrusive positive linkage result in the formula

$$R_2/R_1 = r(\alpha) = 5/\cos\alpha$$

Where
  R_2, the posterior link, is the protrusive radius of curvature of the path of the hinge axis,
  R_1, the anterior link, is the radius of curvature of the palatal concavity, and
  α is the angle between the path of the hinge axis and functional length, L_{MD}, of the mandible in centric relation.

The formula connects the posterior and anterior initial radius of curvature of the guiding curves on the condition that the corresponding link quadrangle (Fig. 11–11) possesses the oscillating angle $\Delta\mu = 23°$. The functional lengths, L_{MD} and L_{MX} (of mandible and maxilla, respectively), do not appear in this formula. This means that the structure of the positive movement of the couple is not influenced by its length. Figure 11–20 shows the link quadrangle of an individual and its computed fixed centrode (*A*) and the superimposed corresponding diagram of a prolonged

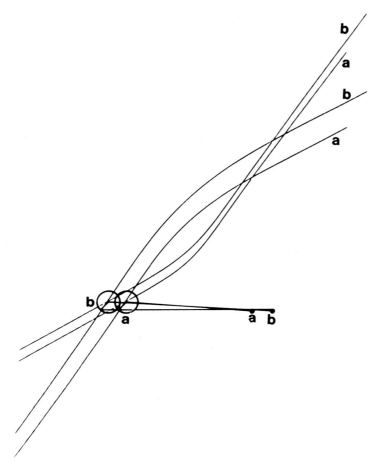

FIGURE 11–20   The fixed centrode as a kinematic invariant of the protrusive gear system. The link quadrangle (a) is plotted in full scale from a patient's data, together with the corresponding fixed centrode of the mandible. The superimposed link quadrangle (b) possesses the same kinematically relevant data (R_2, R_1, and α). Only L_{MD} is prolonged, by about 30 percent. The shape of the fixed centrode is independent of the functional length of the mandible (L_{MD}) (drawing enlarged).

L_{MD} (*B*). The fixed centrodes show the same alignment in space: The kinematic properties of the gear system show no structural variation.

    Conclusion: L_{MD}, the functional length of the mandible, though it is the positively moved couple in the gear system, has no significance for the functioning of the gear system. It describes only the alignment of this system in the skull. Therefore, it is above all a skeletal quantity.

    The analysis of the alignment of L_{MD} in the skull was carried out with 40 individuals. Besides lateral X-rays of the beginning and end of orthodontic treatment, the complete data on the gear systems of these patients were available. The average period of treatment was four years.

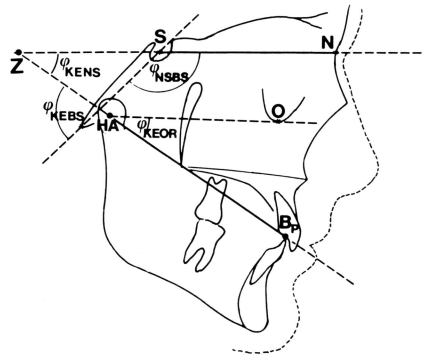

FIGURE 11–21   Couple line (L$_{MD}$) and maxillary angles.

Main results (Fig. 11–21): The couple line L$_{MD}$ is precisely aligned with skeletal structures like the nasion-sella line and the hinge axis-infraorbital line. It can serve as a means by which to analyze the shape of the mandible.

The averages of the angles φ_{KENS} (between L$_{MD}$ and the nasion-sella line) and φ_{KEOR} (between L$_{MD}$ and the hinge axis-infraorbital line) are

$$\varphi_{KENS} = 34.1°, \quad SD = 3.4°$$

$$\varphi_{KEOR} = 30.3°, \quad SD = 2.6°$$

These relatively small standard deviations suggest that both values are features of the sample. The angle φ_{KENS} is scarcely influenced by growth. Table 11–2 shows the simple statistics of the angle differences before and after treatment. The angle φ_{KEOR} is time dependent.

TABLE 11–2   Simple Statistics of the Angle Differences

	Average	*SD*	*t-Test*
φ_{KENS}	0.32°	2.16°	ns
φ_{KEOR}	1.95°	2.84°	p < 0.0001

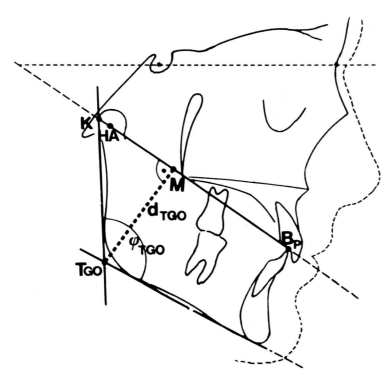

FIGURE 11–22   Couple line (L_{MD}) and mandibular geometrical quantities.

Analysis of the relation between L_{MD} and mandibular structures reveals a high correlation between angle φ_{TGO} and the distance d_{TGO} between L_{MD} and the vertex of the angle φ_{TGO} (FIG. 11–22): r = –0.70. The smaller this distance, the greater is φ_{TGO}. The correlation increases when the influence of only enlargements is eliminated: r = –0.90. This increase (from 0.70 up to 0.90) of the correlation coefficient is extremely statistically significant: p <0.0005.

Interpretation: Since a triangle is defined by three independent factors, the close correlation (–0.90) means that the shape of the mandible is determined only by two quantities: L_{MD} and d_{TGO}. In the interindividual comparison, the couple L_{MD} plays the part of the enlarging factor and the ratio d_{TGO}/L_{MD} that of the shape determining the angle of the mandible (φ_{TGO}). (See references 13 and 14 for further details.)

COUPLE L_{MD} AND GROWTH

ANATOMICAL AND FUNCTIONAL POINTS

The sophisticated analyses of growth done by Bookstein[15] and by Moss[16] make use only of anatomical points. These points are distinguished by morphological features, but Fanghänel[17] has discovered that growth is influenced by a change in function. For example, the growth of rat skulls will be less anisotropic if their forelegs are amputated.

In reference to the findings of Fanghänel, functional points of the visceral cranium, which have a particular biomechanical significance, should be particularly important for growth and therefore for geometric growth analysis. Since the protrusive stomatognathic gear system will function only if the mandibula is pressed to its cranial border by muscular forces, the hinge axis point and the point of inflection of palatinal concavity represent centers of force. The lines of application of the two reactions of support F_1 and F_2, which vectorially add up to the muscular resultant F, run through these points. They are factually given by the ends of L_{MD} in the CO position of the mandibula (Fig. 11–23).

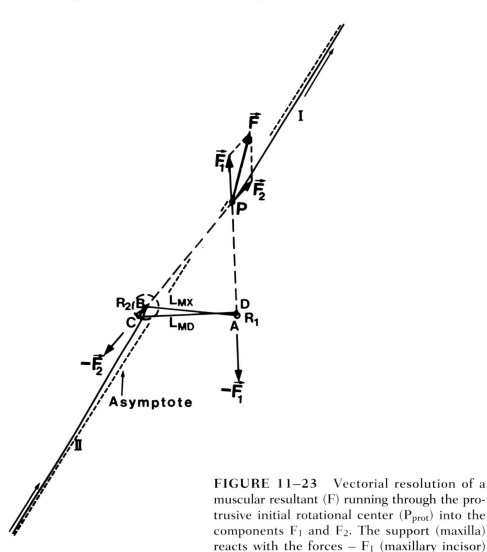

FIGURE 11–23 Vectorial resolution of a muscular resultant (F) running through the protrusive initial rotational center (P_{prot}) into the components F_1 and F_2. The support (maxilla) reacts with the forces $- F_1$ (maxillary incisor) and $- F_2$ (TMJ).

GROWTH SUPERPOSITIONS ON THE LINE OF COUPLE (L_{MD})

One can assume that points on L_{MD} (for example, the force centers) shift by growth along L_{MD}, considering the following findings:

> The kinematics of the protrusive gear system are independent of the length L_{MD}.
>
> L_{MD} plays the part of an enlarging factor in the shaping of the mandible.
>
> The ends of L_{MD} are centers of force.
>
> The angle φ_{KENS} is a sample feature and virtually independent of growth.

Therefore, and also because of the constancy of φ_{KENS}, the nasion sella line and the line of couple, together with their vertex Z, can be used as a coordinate reference system for growth analysis. The nasion sella line, as well as the functional L_{MD} line (arbitrary hinge axis point = assumed center of the condyles and the incisal edge), can be located in lateral X-rays without difficulty. Figure 11–24 paradigmatically shows the tracing of two X-rays of one individual superimposed on the individual's oblique-angled

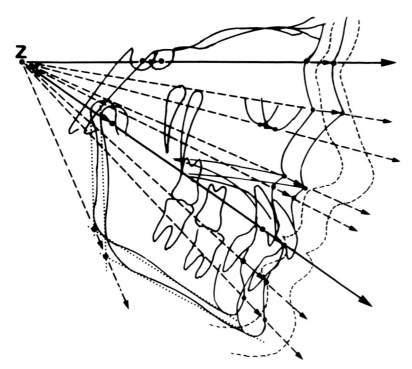

FIGURE 11–24   Superposition of two lateral X-ray pictures of an individual on the L_{MD} line and on the intersection Z of L_{MD} with the nasion sella line.

TABLE 11–3

Angle between Line of Couple and	X-Ray (1)	X-Ray	Difference	t-Value	Significance
Sella	34.0°	33.7°	−0.27°	0.64	ns
Nasion	34.0°	34.0°	+0.04°	0.16	ns
Infraorbital	18.7°	19.6°	+0.90°	3.05	p < 1%
Spina	10.4°	10.2°	−0.20°	1.53	ns
A-point	7.35°	7.46°	+0.11°	0.30	ns
B-point	−9.30°	−9.15°	+0.15°	0.56	ns
Pogonion	−13.4°	−13.1°	+0.35°	1.67	ns
Menton	−16.5°	−16.1°	+0.38°	2.08	p < 5%
TGO point	−32.7°	−32.5°	+0.27°	1.32	ns
Angle between TGO and Z-N	66.5°	66.6°	+0.15°	0.08	ns

coordinate system of nasion sella line and line of couple (time difference: four years). Z seems to be a center of growth for the visceral cranium, which describes almost all cephalometrically important points lying on radial lines. The statistics also confirm this statement. In Table 11–3, the angles between the line of couple and the connecting line are listed for several anatomical points with the center Z. With the exception of the infraorbital point and the menton, all angles remain constant. The constancy of the angle between TGO and Z-N is remarkable. The visceral cranium seems to pour out of this "cone" TGO–Z-N by growth.

The use of biomechanically functional points seems to be a rather successful way of finding an allometric center, at least for practical purposes. This practical utility is confirmed by the fact that for all 40 individuals examined a superimposition (corresponding to the quality of Fig. 11–24) could be carried out. It seems that an allometric center of growth within the visceral cranium can be related to *any individual* by means of functional points. A more exact statistical examination in reference to the studies of Moss[16] and Bookstein[15] cannot be carried out because Moss and Bookstein used *inter*individual group comparisons. But the findings corresponding to Figure 11–24 require *intra*individual comparisons. For that, more than two X-rays of one individual are needed.

CURVE OF SPEE

BIOMECHANICAL ALIGNMENT OF CURVE OF SPEE WITH ANATOMICAL STRUCTURES OF THE VISCERAL CRANIUM

The maxillary curve of Spee was determined as the connecting line of the maxillary foveae starting at the basepoint B_p.[18] The individual curve can be closely fitted by a circle (Fig. 11–25). Its radius, R_K, has almost the

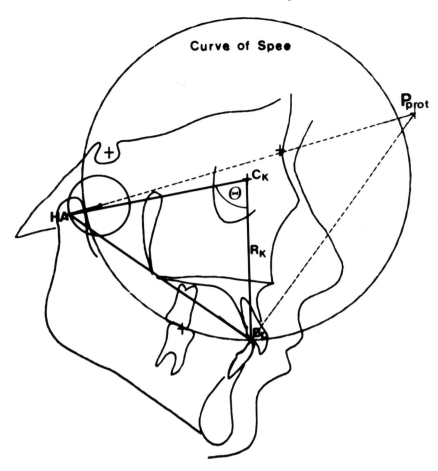

FIGURE 11–25 Curve of Spee fitted by a circle and drawn from an X-ray of an individual. C_K = center; R_K = radius.

same value as the functional length of the mandible L_{MD} (Table 11–4), but the standard deviations are different: SD (R_K) = 3 · SD (L_{MD}). This difference is quite significant (n = 23, F-test: p < 0.001). It means that L_{MD} is an interindividual constant in comparison with R_K, indicating that R_K has no skeletal significance but has a functional significance. The same conclusion yields the measurement of the distance (n) between the center (C_K) of the curve of Spee and the nasion sella line (Fig. 11–26). The variance of the variable n has approximately the same high value as the much longer radius R_K. At the same time n and R_K are very strongly correlated: r

TABLE 11–4 Simple Statistics of R_K and L_{MD}

	Average (mm)	Standard Deviation (mm)
R_K	92	19.5
L_{MD}	96	6.4
n	9	18.8

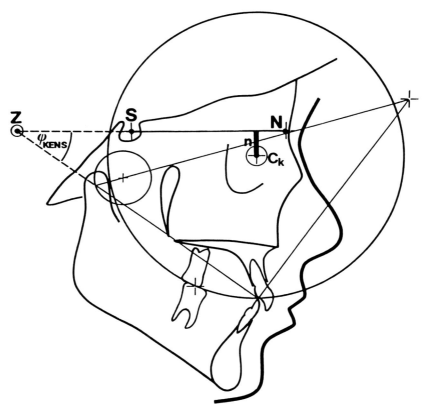

FIGURE 11–26   Curve of Spee and nasion-sella line. n = distance of C_K from the nasion sella line.

$(n, R_K) = 0.96$ (95 percent confidence interval: $0.92/0.985$). This high correlation coefficient is possible only because the substantial individual variation is represented by functional and not by skeletal quantities.

THE PROTRUSIVE GEAR SYSTEM AND THE CURVE OF SPEE

In statistical average the prolonged maxillary circular curve of Spee meets the hinge axis and the protrusive initial center of rotation (P_{prot}) (Fig. 11–25). These findings represent a geometrical triviality when the incisor alignment is ideal.[18] The hinge axis HA, basepoint B_p, and center P_{prot} are positioned on the circle of Thales around C_K. Therefore, the angle HA-C_K-P_{prot} should be 180°. This hypothesis is confirmed by measurement: average = 183°, standard deviation = 25°, N = 23.[18] Individual deviations from the biomechanical ideal, which satisfy a certain law, account for this high standard deviation, as is demonstrated by two cases.

Case I: Figure 11–27 shows the tracing of a lateral X-ray on which the gear parameters are drawn full scale. The incisor alignment deviates

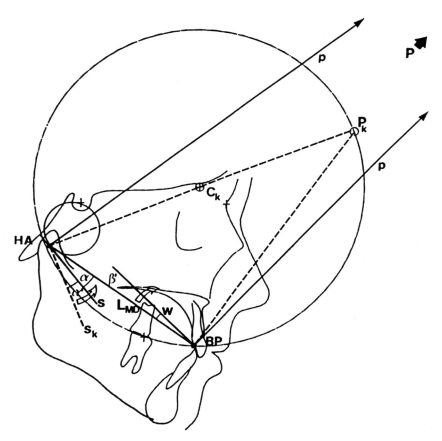

FIGURE 11–27 Compensation mechanism of the inclinations of guidances. See text for details.

from the biomechanical ideal, since the palatal tangent of inflection (w) does not meet the hinge axis (HA) (w and L_{MD} do not coincide). This deviation is recorded by the angle β'. The initial posterior tangent (s) and the anterior tangent (w) define the initial protrusive center of rotation P_{prot} by means of the polar lines (p). In the biomechanical ideal, w and L_{MD} should coincide, the momentary rotational center should be P_k, and the initial tangent of the hinge axis path should be positioned in s_k. In comparison with s_k, s is swiveled through α'.

Case II: Figure 11–28 shows inverse deviations compared with case I.

In conclusion, it seems that compensating rotations of the initial guidances are possible when the momentary rotational center P_{prot} is shifted along a line that coincides with the application line of the resultant force vector of the muscular apparatus that holds the mandibula in centric occlusion. Statistically, the angles α' and β' are correlated by the coefficient $r_{\alpha'\beta'} = 0.61$. Considering the relatively high inexactitude of

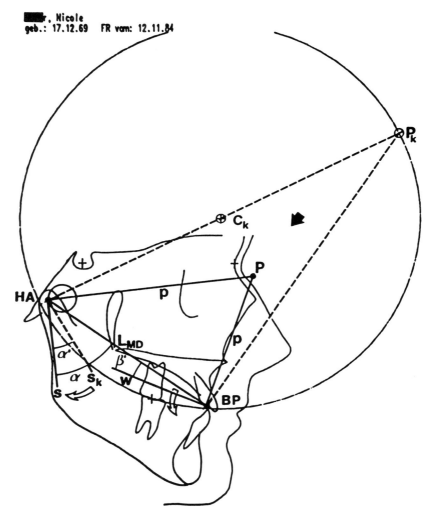

FIGURE 11–28   Compensation mechanism of the inclinations of guidances. See text for details.

measurement of the two angles α' and β' (small differences), this correlation coefficient possesses an unexpectedly high value. The curve of Spee can be considered as the fundamental feature, in whose course the anterior and posterior guidance can simultaneously adapt themselves to the muscular apparatus.

SUMMARY AND OUTLOOK

The stomatognathic system represents a complex machine that is controlled by the instantaneously acting neuromuscular feedback system and by delayed adaptation. An optimal functioning requires an optimal mechanism. Criteria for the biomechanical ideal of the single occlusal elements can be derived from the morphology and mechanical functioning. The theoretical considerations can be confirmed by empiricism and experiment.

But the single ideal arrangement has a different significance. The coincidence of the centric occlusion with the centric relation of the TMJ is more important than the relation of the lower incisal edge to the inflection point of the palatal concavity, the base point (B_p). The relation CO = CR of the TMJ is more significant than the baseline arrangement of the incisors (incisors-joint) because in contrast to the posterior guidance of the TMJ for the retrusive anterior guidance, there is a separate guidance (retrusive-joint of premolars). An anterior position in CO of the incisal contact point is more likely than an anterior position of the condyle out of CR.

Compensating mechanisms follow superior requirements of the entire stomatognathic system. For example, the deviations of the initial inclinations of the anterior and posterior guidance are such that the inclination of the fixed centrode remains almost constant.

Mechanical stability depends upon functional parameters such as the curvatures of the guidances. If the curvature of the short retrusive path of the hinge axis is too small, the result is a retrusive fixed centrode that is too steep. This can cause mechanical instabilities when the mandible is pressed in its cranial borders by the muscles, as can be seen in TMJ cases.

This article includes theoretical considerations. The word "theoretical" is intended according to the spirit of physics that yields no qualitative opinions but falsifiable quantitative individual forecasts—for example, in accordance with the formula $R_2/R_1 = 5/\cos\alpha$ that describes the sound kinematics of the individual mandible.

In this chapter we have analyzed the range of rotation of the mandible. In doing so, we found that with the aid of physical principles we are able to describe not only the movements of the mandible on the cranial borders of the occlusion but also the protrusive gear system, the retrusive gear system, and the gear system of the curve of Spee. The latter, which represents a master gear system, includes the movements of the mandible in the other two gear systems.[18] We found that free mandible movements follow the same physical principles. This means that free mandible moving cycles are neuromuscularly guided gear movements (Fig. 11–29A and B).[19] Computer simulations of the movements of the corresponding gear systems and of the corresponding couple points show that these follow the same paths as that of the mandible. Thus, there is no difference between neuromuscularly free-guided, occlusal-guided, or mixed-guided mandibular movements.

Result: Occlusion and joint structures seem to be neuromuscular movement cycles that became or are meteria.

At the same time, as the foregoing examples have demonstrated, biomechanical analysis is more than a mechanistic way of thinking about the stomatognathic system. We believe that the demands of the neuromuscular

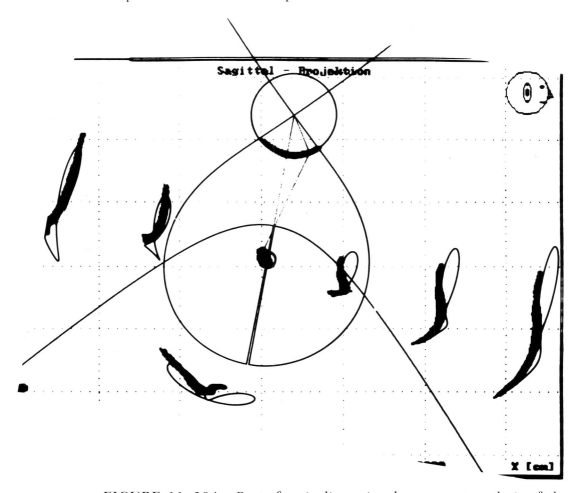

FIGURE 11–29A   Part of a six-dimensional movement analysis of the mandible of a patient. Five cycles of maximal opening and closing are drawn in the midsagittal plane. I = Incisor point; HA= Hinge axis position in CR.
Other curves of points on the ridged mandible body (even outside anatomical structures) can be followed. They allow the practitioner to find and construct the corresponding gear system of maximum opening. The patient's movements are superimposed on the computer plot of the resulting gear system and movement of corresponding couple points. The mandible uses two of the possible four half-cycles.

system and those of biomechanics must be joined in order to guarantee an optimal, functional system. In this sense, the morphological outline of the functional surfaces of the stomatognathic system are the result of and at the same time the basis for an optimal working neuromuscular system.

The material presented here concerns only the cranial border movement in the vicinity of CO. In the future, a primary goal will be to reduce the wide variety of mandibular movements to a few individual constants. It appears as though this objective is feasible, so that the entire range of

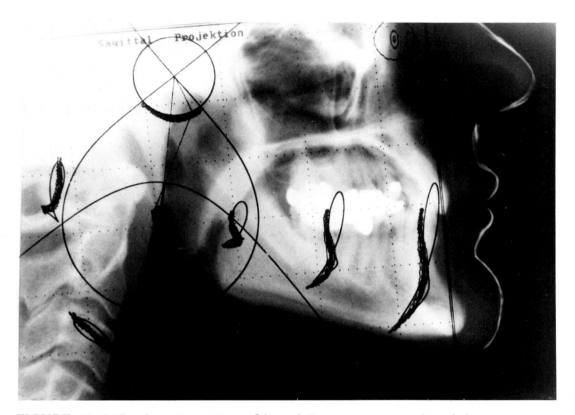

FIGURE 11–29*B* Superimposition of lateral X-ray movement; plot of the patient and corresponding computer plot of the specific gear system with corresponding couple points. The gear system itself has a strong relation to anatomical structures.

mandibular movements can be reduced to a single interlocking gear system in which the same cycles are always used.

As our knowledge of these complex, interdependent systems increases, the hope grows that diagnostic and therapeutic strategies can be developed that yield more long-term stability of orthodontic treatment and help us to understand ongoing changes as the consequence of natural development.

REFERENCES

1. Kubein, D: Die kraniale Grenzfunktion des Stomatognathen Systems des Menschen Hanser, München, 1985.
2. Nägerl H, Kubein-Meesenburg D, Fanghänel J, Berndt A: Retrusive Gelenkfunktion und Stabilitätsbereich der Mandibulla. Dtsch Zahnärztl Z 45:54–58, 1990.

3. Kubein-Meesenburg D, Nägerl H, Fanghänel J: Elements of a general theory of joints. 1. Basic kinematic and static function of diarthrosis. Anat. Anz. 170:301–308, 1990.

4. Schumacher GH: Funktionelle Morphologie der Kaumuskulatur. Jena, VEB Gustav Fischer Verlag, 1961.

5. Motsch A: Spannungsoptische Experimente zur funktionellen Anatomie des Unterkiefers. Habilitationsthesis, Freiburg, 1956.

6. McCollum BB: Fundamentals involved in prescribing restorative dental remedies. *In* McCollum BB, Stuart CE: A research report. Ventura, 1955.

7. McHorris WH: Okklusion unter besonderer Brücksichtigung von Funktion und Parafunktion der Frontzähne. Inf Orthod u Kieferorthop 12:7–44, 1980. Translated in J Clin Orthod 13:606–620, 684–701, 1979.

8. Kubein-Meesenburg D, Nägerl H, Meyer G, Jäger A, Radlanski RJ, Sattler G, Harder, D: Zur okklusalen Morphologie: Vergleich der Konturkurven von Front- und Seitenzähnen. Dtsch Zahnärztl Z 41:21–28, 1986.

9. Nägerl H, Kubein-Meesenburg D: Comparative examination for the determination of the individual contour-curve from the incisors and from the premolar region. Anat Anz 170:163–170, 1990.

10. Kubein-Meesenburg D, Nägerl H, Klamt B: The biomechanical relation between incisal and condylar guidance of man. J Biomech 21:997–1009, 1988.

11. Kubein-Meesenburg D, Nägerl H: The biomechanical law of linkage of anterior and posterior guidance. J Gnatho 8:53–71, 1989.

12. Kubein-Meesenburg D, Nägerl H: Basic principles of relation of anterior and posterior guidance in the stomatognatic system. Anat Anz 171:1–12, 1990.

13. Kubein-Meesenburg D, Nägerl H, Fanghänel J, Schwestka R: Die Anordnung des stomatognathen Koppelsystems im Schädel. Dtsch Zahnärztl Z 44:23–26, 1989.

14. Kubein-Meesenburg D, Nägerl H, Schwestka R, Jäger A: Wachstum des Gesichtsschädels und Biomechanik des Stomatognathen Systems. Inf Orthod Kieferorthop (1) 53–71, 1990.

15. Bookstein FL: The geometry of cranial growth invariants. Am J Orthod 83:221–234, 1983.

16. Moss, ML, Skalak R, Patel H, Sen K, Moss-Salentjin L, Shinozuka M, Vilmann H: Finite element method modelling of craniofacial growth. Am J Orthod 87:453–470, 1985.

17. Fanghänel J: Der Einfluß formgestaltender Faktoren auf das postnatale Wachstum mit besonderer Berücksichtigung der Statik; ein Beitrag zur quantitativen Erfassung von Problemen des Wachstums und der Adaptation. Medical dissertation, (B), University of Rostock, 1974.

18. Kubein-Meesenburg D, Nägerl H, Fanghänel J: Zur Biomechanik der sagittalen Kompensationskurve. Dtsch Zahnärztl Z 45:44–47, 1990.

19. Kubein-Meesenburg D, Nägerl H, Fanghänel J: Die getriebemechanische Beschreibung der Unterkieferbewegung. *In* Oral Anatomie, Rostock. 1990.

Functional Stability of Orthodontic Treatment— Occlusion as a Cause of Temporomandibular Disorders

Arthur T. Storey

Stability of the occlusion may be defined in either structural or functional terms. Structural stability is the criterion used in assessing the presence or absence of postorthodontic relapse. The absence of posttreatment relapse is an indication of structural stability, both occlusal and skeletal. Andrews' Six Keys of Occlusion[1] are examples of structural criteria. Another concept of stability, frequently used in dentistry, is that of good intercuspation, with multiple tooth contacts, so that there are no "slides in centric." This is a statement of functional stability. Functional stability is a criterion used to assess a potential or presumed cause of dysfunction due to a neuromuscular maladaptation. Gnathologically oriented orthodontists emphasize the importance of functional stability in preventing maladaptations to occlusal interferences. Roth[2] has championed functional criteria for an ideal orthodontic occlusion. This chapter discusses both types of stability and their interactions. Two questions are addressed. Can occlusal interferences cause relapse of dental and/or skeletal relationships? and Can occlusal interferences cause temporomandibular disorders?

Responses to occlusal interferences take several forms. In the absence of a reflex response the interfering tooth may be moved out of the offending position. Evidence in support of this assertion comes from an unpublished investigation examining the consequences of a mild working-side interference carried out in the laboratory of Professor Hans Graf in Berne, Switzerland. The hypothesis to be tested was that over a period of several weeks hypernormal biting forces on a mild working-side interference would elicit a reflex avoidance of the interference. The study entailed building up the buccal inclines of the lingual cusps of a lower right first molar crown that had been placed on a postcore preparation. In order to measure the forces on this crown, the occlusal form was duplicated on a three-dimensional sensor described by Graf, Grassl, and Aeberhard.[3] The occlusal table and sensor were placed over the postcore preparation during the experimental sessions. This force transducer recorded forces in three planes (the axial, mesiodistal, and buccolingual) with crosstalk between channels less than 5 percent. Lower incisor position in posture and in chewing and swallowing was monitored in three dimensions by two infrared cameras tracking a light-emitting diode affixed to the lower incisors.[4] Neuromuscular responses to the interference were recorded by electromyography using surface hook electrodes in the temporalis and masseter muscles.[5] The mobility of the tooth with the interference was evaluated at each visit using the periodontometer of Muhlemann.[6] The subject was closely monitored before, during, and after the experiment for signs and symptoms of TMD. The subject was evaluated before (1 day and immediately prior to) insertion of the interference, 6 hours and 2, 9, and 16 days following placement, and 30 days after removal of the interference.

Forces on the first molar during mastication were found to increase slightly in the axial and buccolingual directions during the experiment. There was no evidence of a neuromuscular response to the interference by changes in amplitude, duration, or symmetry of muscle action potentials or by the appearance of silent periods on tooth contact. An absence of any avoidance of the interference was confirmed from the jaw-tracking records. Almost immediately (on day 2) the molar tooth demonstrated increased mobility at displacement forces of both 1 and 5 g. By patient report and use of occlusal contact marking, the interference disappeared—presumably by intrusion. At no time did the patient develop any signs or symptoms of TMD. Conclusions drawn from this investigation on this patient were that

1. The mild working-side interference was not reflexly avoided.
2. The interference did not give rise to any signs or symptoms of TMD.
3. The tooth became mobile and subsequently intruded.

Earlier studies by Schaerer, Stallard, and Zander,[7] using switches recording intercuspal and interference positions, had established that mild working-side interferences were not reflexly avoided—that is, closure into intercuspal position was guided solely by the occlusal inclines. The adaptive response to mild working-side interferences would appear to be by tooth movement. This passive (nonreflex) adaptation is illustrated in Figure 12–1A.

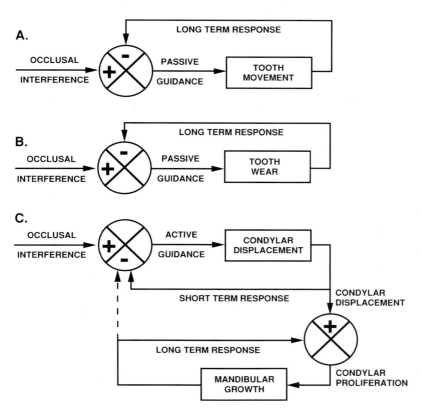

FIGURE 12–1   Occlusal interferences may give rise to passively and actively mediated responses. In the absence of a reflex response during chewing, teeth may move (*A*) or abrade (*B*). When reflex adaptations occur, the mandible shifts to avoid the interference(s) producing condylar displacement(s) (*C*). This active response may lead to condylar cartilage proliferation and mandibular growth in growing animals.[37]

Another passive adaptation that could account for reduction of mild occlusal interferences is wear of the tooth in subjects eating abrasive diets. Figure 12–2 illustrates the extent to which abrasion can reduce tooth structure in persons living on or near deserts. Bread made from stone-ground flour also facilitates tooth wear. Canine guided occlusions gradually become "group function" occlusions due to wear of the maxillary canine. Functional abrasion (in contrast to parafunctional abrasion, as seen in bruxism), while considered normal by anthropologists and paleontologists and crucial to hypotheses of jaw function in ancient man, is considered pathological by gnathologists. (The correspondence between Beverly McCollum and Charles Moses[8] on this controversy makes fascinating reading.) Functional wear is another possible adaptation to occlusal interferences (see Fig. 12–1*B*).

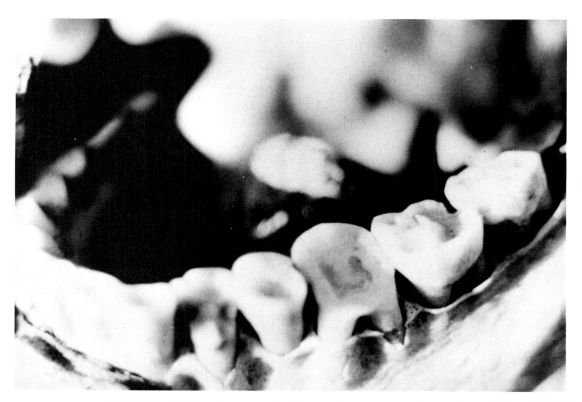

FIGURE 12–2   An example of extensive wear leading to loss of the clinical crowns of mandibular bicuspids and molars, with exposure of the pulp in the molar in a skull of a Nubian of the early dynastic period. Wear of teeth is common in skeletal remains of persons living along the Nile.[38]

In contrast to these passive forms of adaptation to occlusal interferences are the active or reflex responses. It is widely accepted that under certain conditions occlusal interferences are avoided. Such an active response to occlusal interferences resulting in "occlusal instability" is used to explain functional malocclusions—for example, functional posterior and anterior cross bites. It has been claimed that these functional malocclusions will become skeletal malocclusions and therefore should be treated immediately. Evidence for a learned response to occlusal interferences was first clearly demonstrated by Schaerer, Stallard, and Zander.[7] Bridges were constructed with switches in bridge pontics that would signal tooth contact in the intercuspal position and on balancing-side interferences during mastication. Following contact with the balancing interference, muscle activity stopped for about 20 ms ("silent period") followed by asymmetric jaw muscle activity, presumably leading to avoidance of the interference. Forty percent of balancing-side interferences showed silent periods—that is, nearly half of the closures following contact on a balancing-side interference were reflex modulated as a consequence of occlusal feedback. Specifically, on initial contact with the interference, the levator muscles fell silent and then shifted the mandible laterally so as to avoid further contact; the occlusal guidance was active (see Fig. 12–1C). The response to initial contact is unlearned or unconditioned. Following multiple contacts on the interference, the offending contact may be avoided through conditioning.

As mentioned earlier, there is the clinical perception that repeated avoidance of an interference may lead to a skeletal response in growing individuals. Anecdotal evidence appears stronger for functional posterior cross bites becoming skeletal asymmetries than functional anterior cross bites becoming skeletal Class III malocclusions. These adaptations in the skeleton can be visualized in the extension of the cybernetic diagram used to illustrate reflex responses to occlusal interferences (see Fig. 12–1C). Here one sees the interaction between structural and functional instability. *In the absence of neuromuscular adaptation, structural adaptations to occlusal interferences occur in the dentition: With neuromuscular adaptation structural adaptations occur in the skeleton.*

Conclusions that may be drawn from these experiments are that (1) occlusal interferences may result in passive adaptation such as tooth movement or tooth wear, and (2) occlusal interferences may result in active adaptations—that is, condylar displacement(s), with the potential for condylar and fossa remodeling in the growing individual. In answer to question 1, the response is yes—occlusal interferences have the potential to cause relapse of dental relationships and potentially alter skeletal development.

Let us now turn to question 2: Can occlusal interferences cause temporomandibular disorders? Occlusal interferences were once considered to be a major cause of TMD. While some clinicians adhere to this hypothesis, evidence for a multifactorial causation of a spectrum of TMDs has markedly shifted this emphasis over the past decade. While once accepting the primacy of occlusal factors, I now believe that trauma and parafunction are more important in causing TMD. Statements in the ADA President's Report[9] and the Consensus Statement of the American Academy of Pediatric Dentistry[10] strongly de-emphasize an occlusal etiology. Numerous studies (e.g., Droukas, Lindée, and Carlsson[11]) have documented as high a prevalence of occlusal interferences in the asymptomatic population as in patients suffering from TMD. This has led some people to believe that occlusal factors do not play a role, or play only a minor role, in the causation of TMD.

Whereas absent or low correlations between occlusal factors and signs and symptoms of dysfunction indicate a minor role in the etiology of TMD, weaknesses in most of the epidemiological studies need to be recognized and corrected in future studies. Even though multiple etiologies for TMD are now universally acknowledged, most studies have not attempted to segregate patients or subjects so that those of possible occlusal etiology are not greatly outnumbered by those of traumatic and parafunctional etiology. Miettinen[12] in his textbook on occurrence research in medicine stresses the need for examining the subset of the population in which the investigator is looking for associations. He makes the point well, using diabetics as an example: "The clinical epidemiologist, interested in nutrition, studies the occurrence of various complications of adult-onset diabetes in relation to diet *among such diabetics* (author's emphasis), instead of the effects of diet on the risk of diabetes and other states and events of health among people at large." Murphy[13] makes the same observation in regard to orthodontic treatment as a cause of periodontal disease. He states that "to demonstrate clear statistical significance *homogeneous subsets* [author's emphasis] must be used." Parker,[14] in presenting a model for the etiology of TMD, also asserts the need for segregating samples: "As long as TMD populations are not differentiated, etiologies are likely to remain amorphous."

The problems of finding a meaningful association between occlusal interferences and TMD can be seen in the following hypothetical examples. Suppose that in a treatment sample 44 percent of the patients developed the disorder as a result of a parafunction, in 41 percent of the patients the disorder was of traumatic origin, and 15 percent had symptoms due to occlusal interferences (see Fig. 12–3). If the assumption is made that 30 percent of an asymptomatic sample engaged in significant parafunction, that 20 percent had comparable traumatic accidents, and that 5 percent had occlusal interferences, the numbers of subjects needed to demonstrate a significant association can be calculated. (Note that the prevalences do not add up to 100 percent—the prevalences are expected to be lower in the control group.) The power of the association—that is, the likelihood that occlusal interferences are significantly associated with TMD—will be determined by the significance level desired (usually 0.05 or 0.01), the Critical Size Effect, and the number of subjects. For the hypothetical distributions given above, the Critical Size Effect for the variable occlusal interferences is 10 percent (15 percent minus 5 percent). For a one-sided test at the 0.05 significance level and a power of 0.8, 111 patients per group are required (see Table 12–1). To detect a smaller difference in prevalences, say 5 percent, 343 patients per group are required. A higher power, say 0.9, would require even larger numbers of subjects—

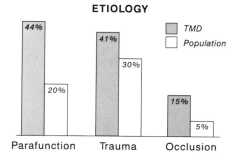

ETIOLOGY

44%   41%   30%   20%   15%   5%

☐ TMD
☐ Population

Parafunction   Trauma   Occlusion

FIGURE 12–3   Estimates of prevalence of parafunction, history of trauma, and occlusal interferences in a hypothetical sample of patients suffering from TMD compared to a hypothetical sample from the general population. The difference in prevalence of occlusal interferences between the two samples is a measure of the Critical Size Effect.[39]

TABLE 12–1   Sample Sizes Required to Demonstrate Differences

TMD SAMPLE	CONTROL SAMPLE	SAMPLE SIZE*	
		$\alpha=.05$, $1-\beta=0.8$	$\alpha=.01$, $1-\beta=0.8$
15%	5%	111	180
15%	10%	343	556

*(One-sided test; data taken from Table 3.1, *Machin and Campbell, 1987.*)

153 per group to detect a 10 percent difference and 474 per group to detect a 5 percent difference. Decreasing the significance level also requires more patients. For example, with a power of 0.8 and a significance level of 0.01, 180 patients per group are required to detect a 10 percent difference between the groups, and 556 are required to detect a 5 percent difference (see Table 12–1). Since the prevalence of occlusal interferences has been reported to be approximately the same in the general population as in the treatment populations, the Critical Size Effect is very small and the number of subjects needed to establish an association is unrealistically high. It is not surprising, therefore, that epidemiological studies, most with inadequate numbers of subjects, have found only weak or no associations between occlusal interferences and TMD. Further investigators should be sensitive to not only significance levels but also the sample size and power of the study design. The book *How Many Subjects?* by Kraemer and Thiemann[15] is an excellent introduction to the subject. The tables of Machin and Campbell[40] are useful in deriving sample sizes. Future investigators looking for an occlusal etiology should also eliminate patients with a history of trauma or parafunctions. The studies of Pullinger and Seligman[16] indicate a history of trauma in 63 percent of patients with disc displacement with reduction and 79 percent without reduction. Estimates of the prevalence of parafunction in TMD subjects range from 40 percent to 97 percent (Lupton,[17] Grieder,[18] Toller,[19] Trenouth[20]). Whereas the potential exists for identifying the real cause-effect relationships between occlusal factors and TMD from epidemiological studies, past studies have not been adequately designed nor have numbers of subjects been large enough to establish such relationships. Another approach to establishing cause-effect relationships is to provoke TMD in asymptomatic subjects.

Provocation studies rule out many of the confounding variables in epidemiological studies by introducing occlusal interferences into normal, healthy subjects and observing the development of signs and symptoms of

TMD. These prospective studies have examined the effects of working-side interferences[21,22] and balancing-side[23–25] interferences. (Because of the current interest in deep bite as a cause of TMD, a prospective study examining the effects of steep incisal guidance warrants investigation.) In these five provocation studies, 32 subjects out of a total of 59 developed signs and symptoms of TMD. Symptoms were so severe in 6 subjects that they were withdrawn from the studies. Two test subjects were still symptomatic six weeks to nine months after the occlusal interferences were removed. Of great interest is the development of signs and symptoms in one of the control subjects: Signs and symptoms persisted for six weeks after receiving a placebo interference. The results of these studies are summarized in Table 12–2. The time frame for the development of symptoms is interesting. In all the studies except that of Plata, Barghi, and Rey[25] symptoms appeared within a few days. In the Plata et al[25] study, symptoms did not appear until three to five months after insertion of the balancing interference (the results of this study are inaccurately reported

TABLE 12–2   Etiology of TM Disorders—Occlusal Provocation Studies

From Storey AT: Orthodontic treatment and temperomandibular function: The etiology of TM disorders. In Carlson DS: Craniofacial Growth Theory and Orthodontic Treatment. Ann Arbor, University of Michigan, Craniofacial Growth Monograph Series, Center for Human Growth and Development, 1990.

INVESTIGATOR(S)	SUBJECTS	DESIGN	INTERFERENCE	SIGNS AND SYMPTOMS
Riise and Sheikholeslam (J. Oral Rehabil 11:325, 1984)	11♂ (24-32 yrs) dental students	pre/during/post comparison	working (.5mm) max. first molar	During - 12 hr - 8 subjects 2 days - 9 subjects (4 withdraw) 1 week - 4 subjects After - 1 week - 0 subjects
Randow, Carlsson, Edlund and Oberg (Odont. Revy 27:245, 1976)	7♂, 1♀ (22-26 yrs) dental students	pre/during/post comparison	working (.25mm) mand. first molar	During - 24 hr - 7 subjects 1-9 days - 6 subjects (muscle pain) 2-7 days - 4 subjects (TMJ pain) After - 9 months - 1 subject
Magnusson and Enbom (Acta Odont. Scand 42:129, 1984)	24♀ (16-34 yrs) dental nurses and hygienists	double blind, test vs. control	bilateral balancing (3mm deviation at incisors) max. first molars	**TEST** During - 8-9 days - 2 subjects (both withdraw) 2 weeks - 7 subjects (headache) - 4 subjects (muscle fatigue) - 3 subjects (pain in face or jaws) - 2 subjects (TMJ clicking) - 1 subject (limited opening) After - 6 weeks - 1 subject **CONTROL** During - 2 subjects (headache) - 1 subject (muscle fatigue) - 1 subject (pain in face or jaws) After - 6 weeks - 1 subject
Rugh, Barghi and Drago (J. Prosthet. Dent 51:548, 1984)	5♂, 5♀ (26-41 yrs) dental students	pre/during/post comparison	unilateral balancing (0.5 to 1mm deviation at incisors) max. or mand. first or second molars	During - 7 days - 1 subject (TMJ pain) 7 & 14 days - 2/4 subjects (masseter tenderness) - 1/4 subject (lateral pterygoid tenderness) - 4/4 subjects (TMJ sensitivity on palpation) (6/10 subjects free of any signs or symptoms; no nocturnal bruxing in any subjects)
Plata, Barghi and Rey (unpublished)	5♂, 1♀ (16-22 yrs) 1 dental student, 4 non-dental students	pre/during comparison	unilateral balancing (1-2mm deviation at incisors) max. or mand. first molars	During - 2 months - 1 subject 3 months - 3 subjects } "tight occlusion" 4 months - 5 subjects

in the abstract). The comment by one of the investigators (Barghi[25]) that symptoms did not develop until subjects started "to fight the interference" suggests that symptoms in their subjects were due to parafunction. Another important aspect of these studies is that the subjects (with the exception of five subjects in the Plata et al[25] study) are dental, hygiene, and dental nursing students. There are problems in using these "convenience" samples because the subjects are not naive and may have received indications of possible outcome from their teachers or peers. While much more powerful in design than the epidemiological investigations, these provocation studies are weakened by not controlling for suggestion: Future provocation studies must be controlled for suggestion. Investigators should also be aware of numerous predisposing factors[26] that can further complicate these studies.

In response to the question, Can occlusal interferences cause temporomandibular disorders? the answer is yes for 50 percent of the subjects in which occlusal interferences are artificially created. (These studies, however, have not been controlled for suggestion and other predisposing factors.) A logical extension of this question regarding etiology is that of orthodontics causing TMDs. Posttreatment, balancing molar interferences have been implicated as a cause by Roth,[27] as have lingually torqued maxillary incisor crowns by Berry and Watkinson.[28] Maxillary bicuspid extractions (supposedly leading to excessive dorsal positioning of the mandible consequent to maxillary incisor retraction) have been claimed as a cause of TMD.[29] Four European[30–32,36] and three North American[33–35] controlled clinical studies indicate that the prevalence of TMDs is the same in patients 1 to 10 years following orthodontic treatment as in the general population (see Table 12–3). The study of Dorph, Solow, and Carlsen[30] on the prevalence of orthodontic treatment in a TMD clinical sample found more orthodontic treatment among TMD cases than in the general population (p ≤0.05). This observation agrees with the less well-controlled studies of Franks[41] and Berry and Watkinson.[28] The finding may be due to the probability that patients seeking TMD treatment are more likely to have sought orthodontic treatment. Franks's statement that "the majority [of the patients] regularly visited their dental practitioner" supports this hypothesis. The study of Janson and Hasund[31] found fewer signs and symptoms of TMD in their nonextraction group compared to their extraction group (p ≤0.05). Anecdotal claims of nonextraction patients being at lesser risk have been made in the literature. Both the study of Gold[33] and that of Dahl et al[36] document fewer self-reported signs of TMD in treated compared to untreated subjects (p ≤0.001–0.05) and no difference in clinically recorded signs and symptoms. Gold speculated that untreated subjects overreported symptoms in the hopes of obtaining orthodontic treatment. While the collective data suggest that prevalence is the same in treatment samples as in nontreatment samples (see totals in Fig. 12–4), the data do not rule out the possibility that these totals are the algebraic sum of some subjects who are developing TMD and some who are recovering from

---

TABLE 12–3   Etiology of TM Disorders—Orthodontic Treatment

From Storey AT: Orthodontic treatment and temperomandibular function: The etiology of TM disorders. In Carlson DS: Craniofacial Growth Theory and Orthodontic Treatment. Ann Arbor, University of Michigan, Craniofacial Growth Monograph Series, Center for Human Growth and Development, 1990.

INVESTIGATOR(S)	SUBJECTS	DESIGN	TYPE OF ORTHODONTIC TREATMENT	RESULTS	**p<.001 *p<.05 others N.S.
Dorph, Solow and Carlsen (Tandlaegebladet 20:789, 1975)	Patient 20 ♂ 85♀ (14-25 yrs.) Control 31 ♂ 79♀ (14-25 yrs.)	prevalence of orthodontic treatment	Royal Dental College, Copenhagen, Denmark (2-3 yrs. post retention)	prevalence patient group - 28.6%* control group - 26.4%*	
Janson and Hasund (Europ. J. Orthodont. 3.173,1981)	Untreated 12 ♂ 18♀ 4 Bicuspid Extraction 15 ♂ 15♀ Non Extractions 15 ♂ 15♀ (x̄ = 21 yrs.)	prevalence of signs and symptoms	University of Bergen, Norway (1-12 yrs post-retention)	non extraction group fewer signs and symptoms compared to extraction and control groups* extraction group higher frequency for mild disturbances, lower frequency for no, moderate and severe disturbances when compared to untreated group	
Larson and Rönnerman (Europ. J. Orthodont. 3.89, 1981)	Activator (A) 5 4Bi, Full Banding (B) 9 2Bi, Upper Arch Only (C) 5 4Bi, Bimax (D) 4 (24-28 yrs.)	prevalence of signs and symptoms	Institute for Postgraduate Dental Education, Jönköping, Sweden (10 yrs. post retention)	Anamnestic Index Clinical Dysfunction Index A - 0 patients A - 2 patients B - 3 B - 3 C - 0 C - 0 D - 3 D - 4	
Gold, (unpublished master's thesis, 1980)	Treated 170 (x̄ = 18.5 yrs.) Untreated 201 (x̄ = 17.3 yrs.)	prevalence of cardinal signs and symptoms	University of Manitoba, Canada (>6 mos. post treatment)	Treated Untreated Joint Sounds 40%/43% 40%/38% Pain 24%**/25% 46%**/30% Limitation of Movement 5%*/37% 13%**/38%	

INVESTIGATOR(S)	SUBJECTS	DESIGN	TYPE OF ORTHODONTIC TREATMENT	RESULTS	**p<.001 *p<.05 others N.S.
Sadowsky and Begole (Am. J. Orthodont. 78.201, 1980)	Treated 29 ♂ 46♀ Untreated 28 ♂ 47♀ (25 to 55 yrs.)	prevalence of signs and symptoms	six Chicago Orthodontists (>10 yrs. post treatment)	Treated Untreated Pain 9 18 Joint Sounds 23 26 Parafcn. 26 32 CO-CR Shift (lat.) 6 14	
Sadowsky and Polson (Am. J. Orthodont. 86.386, 1984)	Treated Illinois Eastman 96 ♂ 111♀ (x̄ = 39 yrs.) (x̄ = 29 yrs.) Untreated Illinois Eastman 103 ♂ 111♀ (x̄ = 38 yrs.) (x̄ = 33 yrs.)	prevalence of signs and symptoms	University of Illinois and Eastman Dental Center (>10 yrs. post retention)	TMJ Sounds Illinois 34% 42% Eastman 32% 29% Pain Illinois 15% 21% Eastman 16% 15%	
Dahl, Krogstad, Øgaard and Eckersberg (Acta Odontol. Scand. 46.89-93, 1988)	Treated 23 ♂ 28♀ Untreated 28 ♂ 19♀ (19 Yrs.)	prevalence of signs and symptoms	three orthodontists in Raufoss, Norway (5 yrs post treatment)	Anamnestic Index Clinical Dysfunction Index Treated Untreated Treated Untreated symptom free symptom free 29.4%* 8.5% 29.4% 46.8% mild symptoms mild symptoms 70.6%* 91.0% 43.1% 40.4% moderate symptoms 27.5% 12.8%	

TMD (see "Worse" and "Better" in Fig. 12–4). As in the general population, some patients can be expected to develop TMDs. While orthodontic treatment may precipitate TMDs, it is important to remember that other factors may predispose the patient to TMD, whereas other factors can perpetuate TMD.[42] In order to clearly identify orthodontic treatment as a cause of TMD it will be necessary to follow orthodontic cases prospec-

INCIDENCE OF TMD (HYPOTHETICAL)
(Epidemiological Studies/Longitudinal)

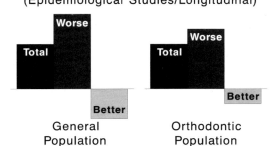

FIGURE 12–4   Epidemiological studies have shown the prevalence of TMD to be similar in patients who have received orthodontic treatment compared to the general population. Were these subjects to be followed longitudinally, it is postulated that the totals will be made up of subjects developing symptoms and subjects recovering from TMD. The proportions of those getting worse and those getting better need not be the same for both the treatment and control samples.

tively. The known cyclic pattern of TMDs is a complication also in need of control. Careful monitoring of trauma and parafunction as initiators during and after treatment will also be necessary.[42]

Acknowledgment: The author is grateful for the statistical insights and counsel of Dr. George Barnwell in the sections related to study design.

REFERENCES

1. Andrews LF: The six keys to normal occlusion. Am J Orthod 62:296–309, 1972.
2. Roth RH: Functional occlusion for the orthodontist. Part III. Angle Orthod 15:174–198, 1981.
3. Graf H, Grassl H, Aeberhard HJ: A method for measurement of occlusal forces in three directions. Helv Odont Acta 18:7–11, 1974.
4. Joss A, Graf H: A method for analysis of human mandibular occlusal movement. Helv Odont Acta 89:1211–1241, 1979.
5. Ahlgren J: Mechanism of mastication: A quantitative cinematographic and electromyographic study of masticatory movements in children, with special reference to occlusion of the teeth. Acta Odontol Scand 24 (Suppl 44):1–109, 1966.
6. Muhlemann HR: Periodontometry, a method of measuring tooth mobility. Oral Surg 4:1220–1233, 1951.
7. Schaerer P, Stallard RE, Zander HA: Occlusal interferences and mastication: An electromyographic study. J Prosthet Dent 17:438–449, 1967.
8. Postgraduate Education. A compilation of articles, papers, lectures and essays by Beverly B. McCollum, DDS. *In* Oral Rehabilitation and Occlusion, Vol. III. San Francisco, University of California, School of Dentistry, 1972, pp. 1–38.
9. Laskin D, Greenfield W, Gale E, Rugh J, Neff P, Alling C, Ayer WA: The President's Conference on the Examination, Diagnosis and Management of Temporomandibular Disorders. Am Dent Assoc 1983, pp.1–84.
10. American Academy of Pediatric Dentistry. Treatment of temporomandibular disorders in children: Summary statements and recommendations. J Am Dent Assoc 120:265–269, 1990.

11. Droukas B, Lindée C, Carlsson GE: Relationship between occlusal factors and signs and symptoms of mandibular dysfunction: A clinical study of 48 dental students. Acta Odontol Scand 42:277–283, 1984.

12. Miettinen OS: Theoretical Epidemiology: Principles of Occurrence Research in Medicine. New York: John Wiley, 1985.

13. Murphy NC: Letter to the editor. Am J Orthod Dentofacial Orthop 94:264, 1988.

14. Parker, MW: A dynamic model of etiology in temporomandibular disorders. J Am Dent Assoc 120:283–290, 1990.

15. Kraemer HC, Themann S: How Many Subjects? Statistical Power Analysis in Research. Newbury Park, CA, Sage Publications, 1987, pp.1–120.

16. Pullinger A, Seligman D: Association of TMJ diagnostic subgroups with general trauma and MVA. J Dent Res 67:403 (abstr), 1988.

17. Lupton DE: A preliminary investigation of the personality of female temporomandibular joint dysfunction patients. Psychother Psychosom 14:199–216, 1966.

18. Grieder A: Psychologic aspects of prosthodontics. J Prosthet Dent 30:736–744, 1973.

19. Toller P. Non-surgical treatment of dysfunctions of the temporo-mandibular joint. Oral Sci Rev 1:70–85, 1976.

20. Trenouth MJ: The relationship between bruxism and temporomandibular joint dysfunction as shown by computer analysis of nocturnal tooth contact patterns. J Oral Rehabil 6:81–87, 1979.

21. Riise C, Sheikholeslam A: Influence of experimental interfering occlusal contacts on the activity of the anterior temporal and masseter muscles during mastication. J Oral Rehabil 11:325–333, 1984.

22. Randow K, Carlsson K, Edlund J, Öberg T: The effect of an occlusal interference on the masticatory system: An experimental investigation. Odont Revy 27:245–256, 1976.

23. Magnusson T, Enbom L: Signs and symptoms of mandibular dysfunction after introductions of experimental balancing-side interferences. Acta Odontol Scand 42:129–135, 1984.

24. Rugh JD, Barghi N, Drago CF: Experimental occlusal discrepancies and nocturnal bruxism. J Prosthet Dent 51:548–553, 1984.

25. Plata M, Barghi N, Rey R: Clinical evaluation of induced occlusal dysharmonies. J Dent Res 61–204 (abstr), 1982.

26. Friction JR, Kroening RJ, Hathaway KM: TMJ and Craniofacial Pain: Diagnosis and Management. St Louis, MO, Ishiyaku EuroAmerica, Inc., 1988.

27. Roth RH: Temporomandibular pain-dysfunction and occlusal relationships. Angle Orthod 32:136–153, 1973.

28. Berry DC, Watkinson AC: Mandibular dysfunction and incisor relationship. A theoretical explanation of the clicking joint. Br Dent J 144:74–7, 1978.

29. Farrar WB, McCarty WL: A Clinical Outline of the Temporomandibular Joint Diagnosis and Treatment. Montgomery, AL, Walker Printing Company, 1983.

30. Dorph G, Solow B, Carlsen O: Fejlfunktion i mastikationssystemet efter orthodontibehandling? Tandlaegebladet 79:789–792, 1975.

31. Janson M, Hasund A: Functional problems in orthodontic patients out of retention. Eur J Orthod 3:173–179, 1981.

32. Larsson E, Rönnerman A: Mandibular dysfunction symptoms in orthodontically treated patients ten years after the completion of treatment. Eur J Orthod 3:89–94, 1981.

33. Gold PL: The Role of Orthodontic Treatment and Malocclusion in the Etiology of Mandibular Dysfunction. Thesis, Department of Preventive Dental Science, University of Manitoba. 1980.

34. Sadowsky C, BeGole EA: Long-term status of temporomandibular and functional occlusion after orthodontic treatment. Am J Orthod 78:201–212, 1980.

35. Sadowsky C, Polson AM: Temporomandibular disorders and functional occlusion after orthodontic treatment: Results of two long-term studies. Am J Orthod 86:386–390, 1984.

36. Dahl BL, Krogstad BS, Ogaard B, Eckersberg T: Signs and symptoms of craniomandibular disorders in two groups of 19 year old individuals, one treated orthodontically and the other not. Acta Odontol Scand 46:89–93.

37. Storey AT, Kenny DJ: Growth, development, and aging of orofacial tissues: Neural aspects. Adv Dent Res 3(1):14–29, 1989.

38. Storey AT: The Diet and Dentition of New Kingdom Pharaohs. *In* Anderson DJ, Matthews B (eds): Mastication. Bristol, England, John Wright & Sons Ltd., 1976, pp. 5–15.

39. Storey AT: Orthodontic treatment and temporomandibular function: The etiology of TM Disorders. *In* Carlsson DS (ed.): Craniofacial Growth Theory and Orthodontic Treatment. Craniofacial Growth Series 23. Ann Arbor, MI, Center for Human Growth and Development, University of Michigan, 1990, pp. 105–115.

40. Machin D, Campbell MJ: Statistical Tables for the Design of Clinical Trials. Oxford, England, Blackwell Scientific Publications, 1987.

41. Franks AST: The dental health of patients presenting with temporomandibular joint dysfunction. Br J Oral Surg 5:157–166, 1967.

42. McNeill C (ed): Craniomandibular Disorders—Guidelines for Evaluation, Diagnosis, and Management. Chicago, Quintessence Publishing Co., 1990.

INDEX

Note: Page numbers in *italics* indicate illustrations; those followed by t refer to tables.